CURE
CODEPENDENCY AND
CONQUER
AS AN EMPATH

How to Break the Codependency Cycle Once and For All By using The Ultimate Guide Through Self Healing and Recovery from Narcissistic Relationships, Self Esteem

Teresa Williams Dr Miller Scarlett

© Copyright 2020 by Teresa Williams Dr Miller Scarlett

All rights reserved.

The material contained herein is presented with the intent of furnishing pertinent and relevant information and knowledge on the topic with the sole purpose of providing entertainment. The author should thus not be considered an expert on the topic in this material despite any claims to such expertise, first-hand knowledge and any other reasonable claim to specific knowledge on the material contained herein. The information presented in this work has been researched to ensure its reasonable accuracy and validity. Nevertheless, it is advisable to consult with a duly licensed professional in the area pertaining to this topic, or any other covered in this book, in order to ensure the quality and validity of the advice and/or techniques contained in this material.

This is a legally binding statement as deemed so by the Committee of Publishers Association and the American Bar Association in the United States. Any reproduction, transmission, copying or otherwise duplication of the material contained in this work are in violation of current copyright legislation. No physical or digital copies of this work, both total and partial, may not be done without the Publisher's express written consent. All additional rights are reserved by the publisher of this work.

The data, facts and description of events forthwith shall be considered as accurate unless the work is deemed to be a work of fiction. In any event, the Publisher is exempt of responsibility for any use of the information contained in the present work on the part of the user. The author and Publisher may not be deemed liable, under any circumstances, for the events resulting from the observance of the advice, tips, techniques and any other contents presented herein.

Given the informational and entertainment nature of the content presented in this work, there is no guarantee as to the quality and validity of the information. As such, the contents of this work are deemed as universal. No use of copyrighted material is used in this work. Any references to other trademarks are done so under fair use and by no means represent an endorsement of such trademarks or their holder.

TABLE OF CONTENTS

Introduction 1

Chapter 1: The Foundations That Lead To Codependent Relationships 3

    What Is Codependency? 4
    The Love Attitude Scale 7
    To The Codependent, This Is A Strategy 7
    The Struggles When You're A Codependent 10
    Codependency Is *Not* Dependent Personality Disorder (Dpd) 11
    Why Identifying Unhealthy Love Matters 15

Chapter 2: Why Codependent Relationships Are Never Healthy 20

    The Mind And It's Duality 20
    Codependency Is Living In A World Of Denial 22
    You Lose Your Sense Of Value 24
    Love Is Never Unhealthy 29
    Toxic Relationships Will Never Be Good For You .. 32

Chapter 3: Eleven Key Symptoms To Look For And How To Recover 37

    What Are The Eleven Key Signs? 38
    You Need To Learn To Say "No" 47
    You Are Not The Bad Guy For Saying No 49

Chapter 4: Why Narcissistic Partners Seek To Manipulate You 53

    Who Is A Narcissist Anyway? 53

What Does This Mean If I'm In A Relationship
With A Narcissist?...55
The Signs You're Dating A Narcissist.......................56
Why Do They Seek To Manipulate You? 65

Chapter 5: Codependency And Pathological
Loneliness: Why We Stay With Narcissists 69

Understanding Loneliness 70
Understanding Why You Feel Alone 74
Why We Stay With A Narcissist 78

Chapter 6: Identifying Toxic Relationships 85

What Is A Toxic Relationship? 85
A Toxic Relationship Could Be With Anyone 86
The Early Signals 88
Can You Rid Yourself Of These Toxic Personalities?
....97

Chapter 7: The True Feelings Of An Empath 102

What It Means To Be An Empath...........................102
The Advantages Of Being An Empath 105
How An Empath Is Different From Being
Codependent 110

Chapter 8: Begin Breaking The Codependency Spell. 119

Finally Breaking Free...120

Love Yourself Enough To Do What Is Right.........133

Chapter 9: Steps To Redraw Boundaries And
Rebuild Relationships ....

Reasons Why You *Need* To Enforce Boundaries ..136
How To Set Healthy Boundaries 145

Chapter 10: Being Comfortable In Your Own Skin....151

    You Don't Live To Live Up To Someone Else's Expectations..152
    How To Stop Caring About What Other People Think..154
    Ditch The Social Media Addiction.........................156
    Start Meditating And Self-Reflecting 158
    Don't Take Things Personally................................161
    You Don't Need Other People To Tell You What You Are Worth 163

Chapter 11: Things You Can Do To Help Yourself....166

    Being Alone Is Not A Bad Thing 167
    How To Be Comfortable Being Alone 175

Chapter 12: Cultivate A Healthy Relationship 182

    Communication Is The Ultimate One 182
    Practice Forgiveness 183
    Understanding The Five Languages Of Love.........187
    Respect Each Other 188
    Be Honest, Open, And Sincere 189
    Appreciate The Ones You Love 192
    Solve Problems Together 193
    Laughter Is Ultimately The Best Medicine.............194
    Make It A Point To Spend Time Together 195

Conclusion 197

INTRODUCTION

Congratulations on purchasing *Cure Codependency* and thank you for doing so.

Codependency is *not a healthy relationship.* But then again, some part of you already knew this. That is why you're reading this book right now. You know that there is something not quite right. Deep down, you know that there is a reason you're struggling to hold on to happiness, and that reason is probably because you are codependent. A codependent relationship can exist in any dynamic. It could be among your friends, family, spouses, and romantic partners. A codependent relationship is when you come to rely so heavily on one person that you believe your world would fall apart without them.

There are several reasons that contribute to why codependency will never be a healthy relationship dynamic. We're going to explore those reasons in the next few Chapters of this book and take a deep dive to understand what codependency is. It is important to break out of this habit and cure yourself once and for all, because relying heavily on one person (or perhaps a couple of people) to get you through life is *never* the way to go. Hinging your happiness on something external will never be the path to achieve lasting happiness. At the end of the day, isn't that what we all want? Every single person in this world *longs* to be happy, and it is one of the many reasons why we form connections in our lives.

Relationships are supposed to bring happiness, but they are never supposed to be the sole source of your happiness. Codependency stems from a root fear of being alone. Loneliness is something nobody wants, and for a codependent person, being with *anyone* is better than the prospect of being alone. This means a codependent is more likely to get into unhealthy relationships and stay in those relationships because they are terrified of being alone.

You *don't* need to stay in a dysfunctional relationship. You don't have to continue in this unhealthy relationship cycle. There is a way to break out of this codependent cycle, and you are now about to discover the answers that you seek.

There are plenty of books on this subject on the market, thanks again for choosing this one! Every effort was made to ensure it is full of as much useful information as possible, please enjoy!

CHAPTER 1

The Foundations That Lead To Codependent Relationships

Are you in a codependent relationship? That could be a question that is difficult to answer unless you know precisely what constitutes a codependent relationship. We all long to fall in love, but what happens when we fall in love with someone who might not be the best fit for us? What happens when we fall for someone who brings out the worst bits about ourselves? How do we differentiate between a love that is healthy and one that is, well, unhealthy?

When you think of a child, family members, close friends, romantic partners, and spouses, the first word that springs to mind is "love." You love these people and you would do anything in the world for them just to see them smile. There are a lot of other emotions associated with these different groups of people in your life too. Trust, security, happiness, excitement, joy, and occasional disappointment and sadness. Love, as they say, is a many-splendored thing. Yet, despite how important love is and what a crucial role it plays in our lives and our happiness, it is interesting that we were never taught explicitly how to love. More importantly, no one ever taught us what it means to cultivate a loving relationship that also happens to be healthy. We navigate the ins and outs of the different relationships in our lives, making mistakes, and figuring it out as we go. One of those mistakes? Not realizing when that love has become unhealthy and led to codependency.

What Is Codependency?

In any healthy relationship, you should be able to depend on the other person. This includes friendships, relationships with your family, and relationships with your partner and spouses. For the relationships that matter, you know that you can depend on the other person to have your back when you need it. You can count on them to lend a helping hand when times are tough, be a shoulder to cry on, and be the support system that you need to help you weather the challenging moments in your life. But when does it cross the line? When do you become *too dependent* on each other to the point that it becomes an unhealthy relationship dynamic? When you start to rely on someone else for *everything*, including your emotional health and your sense of identity, that is when you have crossed the line into the codependent territory.

Hollywood might romanticize the notion of codependency sometimes, but there is nothing healthy about this relationship dynamic. Codependency is a behavior that can be developed because of your desire to be approved of or loved. It is a dysfunctional relationship, and it is not healthy, no matter what your intentions may be. Codependency is unhealthy because it enables or supports one partner's poor behavioral tendencies, such as poor mental health, irresponsibility addiction, underachievement, or immaturity. Codependency essentially means that one person in that relationship is enabling their partner to continue indulging in behaviors that do not contribute to a healthy relationship dynamic. For example, if you were in a relationship with someone who was addicted to gambling. Instead of getting your partner the help that they need to put a stop to their gambling habits, you scramble and try to earn more money because you're trying to make sure you and your partner have enough. With that extra money, your partner then spends it on gambling again, and the unhealthy cycle will continue because neither partner is doing anything about it.

Sometimes, codependency is called *relationship dependency, emotional dependency,* or *obsessive love.* When one person has become so dependent on another for their emotional needs, they often don't feel "complete" without this other person in their life. Whether you're the codependent one or the enabler in the relationship, the one thing you can be sure of is that codependency is unhealthy either way. It is unhealthy because it could lead to habits that end up harming and disrespecting the people that you love. It could be in the form of subtle behaviors where you guilt your friend or partner into spending time with you or making your child feel bad if they didn't get the grades that you hoped they would in school. Perhaps you start sneaking a peek at your partner's texts and emails, worried that they might find someone else and leave you high and dry. You can't imagine your life without them and you become paranoid they are going to walk out the door any second. Part of being human means we can be equally guilty of either behavior. We could be guilty of being on the receiving end of unhealthy relationship behaviors because we enable them, or we could be equally guilty of exhibiting these unhealthy behaviors ourselves.

Codependents are misguided into believing their actions are the only way for them to get what they want. They think that by behaving this way, it is the only way they are going to get the love and support that they crave from the relationships they have. Sadly, codependents don't realize that their behavior is doomed to fail since this approach is never going to lead to a satisfying relationship. This is why the codependent will often end up feeling depressed, stressed, anxious, and eternally unhappy, bouncing from one relationship to the next but always feeling like there is an empty hole or void that needs to be filled.

The Love Attitude Scale

Unlike other related conditions or traits, codependency is not something that a person can be clinically diagnosed with. Instead, codependency is measured by something called *The Love Attitude Scale.* Psychologists used this scale in the late 1990s to help them determine how someone felt about a relationship in their life. In this survey, individuals were asked to think about their partner (or hypothetical one if they were single). They were then asked to either agree or disagree with statements. An example of this statement would be something like this: *When I feel ignored by my partner, I sometimes resort to unreasonable behavior to get their attention.*

Participants were assessed on whether they were codependent or not based on how they scored within a certain range.

To the Codependent, This Is A Strategy

What many people fail to realize is that codependents treat this approach is a strategy. To them, this is a genuine way of getting their needs met, and they don't know any other way to do it. They truly don't realize how flawed this strategy is, because to them, they don't know that their expectations are unrealistic. They genuinely don't realize that the relationship rules and expectations they have set for themselves are unrealistic.

A codependent person is disassociated with themselves. They lack confidence, suffer from low self-esteem and low self-worth, and somewhere in their subconscious mind, they believe that they are unworthy of love. To them, being codependent is the only strategy they know how to use. This is the only lifeline they have of coping because they don't know any other way to do it. They don't know what a healthy relationship looks like. To try and distract themselves from the internal struggles and problems they are silently battling, they rely on the relationships they have in their life to get them through it. They have anxiety and boundary issues when it comes to intimacy and separation from their loved ones. To the codependent, they have a distorted view of the world of relationships.

Some common behaviors a codependent person might exhibit while they are in a relationship include any of the following:

- Anxiety
- Stress and stress-related illnesses
- Hypervigilance
- Compulsion
- Depression
- Excessive reliance
- Denial
- Inability to control their emotions
- Substance abuse

The problem with codependents is that they sometimes allow themselves to remain in a relationship that could be abusive without seeking help because they don't want to be alone. If you do identify with any of the traits above and suspect that you might be suffering from codependency, the next natural question would be, *why am I like this?* Well, the primary root cause of this problem boils down to a disassociation of self. When we don't feel connected to who we are, we struggle to find our sense of self and purpose. When you don't have a sense of self, you seek comfort and support externally, therefore becoming codependent on another.

Codependency is a condition that can be related to depression, anxiety, and stress. This is because when you link your sense of self-worth to someone else, you may feel a need to prove yourself. You end up sacrificing too much to try and make someone else happy, your health included. There is no winner in this type of relationship. Being codependent is a dangerous position to put yourself in, especially if you are in an abusive relationship. When you start believing that on some level, you deserve the abuse that you are being subjected to, you need to seek help. *You never deserve any kind of abuse at the hands of another. NO ONE does.*

The Struggles When You're A Codependent

When you're codependent, you harbor certain belief systems that keep you trapped in this unhealthy cycle. For one thing, you believe that you should never express your thoughts or opinions in a relationship because you believe they are either bad or wrong. You don't believe that your needs are worthy enough, and as a result, you bend over backward trying to please the other people in your life. You prefer to focus all your attention on your partner, or another relationship in your life that you feel strongly about, as a distraction from thinking about your own needs that are not being met. It comes as no surprise that some codependents are people-pleasers, and they don't understand the concept of boundaries. It goes without saying that codependents have no boundaries themselves, or even if they did, they have no idea how to enforce it.

Another struggle of being codependent is that a codependent will hardly ever speak up for themselves. One of the reasons behind this is because they harbor a strong fear of losing the relationship, and because of that, they don't want to risk anything that would make their partner (or anyone else for that matter) feel upset. The people-pleasing tendency in them tells them that they must never say "no" to a request, or risk possibly losing that relationship they are clinging on to forever. They believe that if they lose the relationships they have, they will be alone forever, and those relationships can never be replaced. A codependent sometimes goes out of their way to try and make other people happy at the expense of their own happiness, and this is one of the biggest reasons why they feel unhappy deep down inside. This kind of unhappiness is not going to go away so easily as long as they continue to neglect their needs, desires, and more importantly, neglect what makes them happy.

Codependents are good people. They simply have a bad operating system when it comes to relationships. To initiate the change you want to see in your relationships, you need to change the rules that you follow, and this is why you've decided to pick this book to help you through the process.

Codependency Is *Not* Dependent Personality Disorder (DPD)

The DPD is classified in the Diagnostic and Statistical Manual of Mental Disorders (DSM-5). The DSM-5 is a manual used by clinical psychologists to diagnose their patients. When someone is struggling with DPD, that person feels powerless and incapable of caring for themselves. Someone who is codependent, however, *thinks* that they can function and be fine if they had to be independent. Not necessarily true, but this thought is one of the differentiating factors that set them apart from those who have DPD. Those with DPD are at a greater risk of depression when the relationship they have been holding on to comes to an end.

Those who struggle with DPD struggle to take care of themselves. In fact, their greatest fear is that they *cannot* take care of themselves, and that is why they cling so strongly to certain relationships in their lives. Therefore, they tend to seek everything they need, from care, reassurance, and more, from certain relationships that they have. Those who struggle with DPD generally rely on one main person that they cannot seem to function without. They don't make decisions without this person. They wait for this person to say it is okay to do something before they do it. They won't do anything without this person. They lack self-confidence in such an extreme way that they are unable to think for themselves, hence they rely on this one primary person for everything. For this one who is struggling with DPD, this is an extremely scary way to live. They literally have no idea what they would do if they lost this person. Could you imagine being so terrified and paralyzed by that thought? Imagine going through life believing that you have no idea how to take care of yourself.

A person who has been clinically diagnosed with DPD will identify with the following traits:

- *Struggles to make daily decisions without excessive advice or reassurance from others.*

- *They need others to assume responsibility for a lot of major areas of their life.*

- *They struggle disagreeing with others because they are worried about a loss of support or approval.*

- *When they lose this primary person, they immediately go into panic mode. They feel terrified, unsure of what to do, and it becomes completely chaotic in their mind.*

- *They struggle to initiate independent projects without this primary person they rely on.*

- *They resort to excessive measures at times to attain support from the primary person.*

- *They will put themselves in situations that make them uncomfortable just to accommodate their primary person's needs, wants, and likes.*

- *When they are alone, they feel helpless and uncomfortable.*

- *They suffer from exaggerated fears of being unable to care for themselves.*

It's hard being someone who lives with DPD. Codependency may display some similar tendencies, but ultimately, it is not as severe a condition as DPD is. With DPD, you immediately feel the need to latch on to someone else in your life if you happen to lose the primary person you rely on. When you're living with DPD, the very idea of being alone is something you cannot tolerate. A codependent person might not want to be alone either, but they can still function through the sadness and misery of not having a special relationship in their life that they can turn to. This is not the case with the DPD individual, who will become paralyzed and unable to function once they don't have this primary person in their life.

A codependent person might lack self-confidence, but at least they still have a little bit of it. Someone with DPD has no confidence at all, and this is the reason behind their intense fear of being alone. They have *zero* confidence in their own skills and abilities, and they have no belief in themselves either. Without self-confidence, it becomes easier to see the worst qualities than it is to see the good things you can do. In some extreme cases, poor self-esteem can even lead to feelings of depression and anxiety. They cling tightly to relationships the same way a young child who is unable to care for themselves would.

What DPD and codependents do share in common is that they put themselves at risk of surrounding themselves with negative people (whether knowingly or unknowingly). They apologize even when it's not their fault. It's an unhealthy habit that those with low self-esteem tend to do. A DPD person might give in to their fears and get stuck in that zone of believing they "can't" do something. They believe that they are going to fail, even before they've tried. Past failures have shaken their confidence and they believe this cycle is going to happen again and again. DPD and codependency is a very real problem that a lot of people struggle with day in and day out. There might be times in your life when the symptoms of DPD are going to overlap your codependent tendencies, but that does not necessarily mean you have DPD. You're only guaranteed to have DPD if you have been clinically diagnosed by a professional, and if you feel that you would be more comfortable seeking reassurance from a professional about your condition, you don't have to hesitate. Always seek help when you need it.

Why Identifying Unhealthy Love Matters

The first step to fixing any problem is to realize that there is a problem that needs fixing. Codependency is a form of unhealthy love, and if you don't realize you're in a codependent relationship, you would not have the faintest idea of how to begin overcoming it. How do you identify when the love in your relationship has veered into the unhealthy territory? If any of these signs are present, it's an indication that your relationship might not be as healthy as you thought it was:

- **The Relationship Is Too Intense** - All relationships start off exciting and exhilarating. This applies mostly to romantic relationships and perhaps some friendships too. You revel in each other's company, and the rush of emotion and excitement feels good. Nothing wrong with that, right? Until it shifts from exciting to overwhelming. Perhaps even suffocating, because one person in the relationship can't bear to be away from you for even five minutes. When one person in the relationship begins texting and calling far too often, showing up everywhere you go, wanting to know what you're up to and following you everywhere, impatient when you don't respond quickly despite knowing that you're busy, that relationship has evolved into an unhealthy dynamic. If you don't pay attention to the way that you feel in the early stages of the relationship, it is easy to miss these warning signs.

- **You Don't Have A Chance to Talk About Your Own Needs** - How often do you voice your opinions? How often do you get the opportunity to talk about your own needs in the relationship? Or are you the party that gives, and gives, and gives even more, but receives barely anything in return? Does the other person in the relationship respect your requests? If you're doing all the giving in your relationships, that's another indicator that this dynamic is not the healthiest one to be in.

- **You're Isolated** - This is one of the easiest unhealthy relationship signs that gets overlooked a lot. Isolation begins to creep in one when one person in the relationship starts pulling you away from all the other relationships in your life. For example, if your unhealthy and perhaps codependent relationship was romantic, your partner could be pulling you away from all the other relationships in your life, and you probably don't even realize it. They express an intense desire to want to spend time with you all the time, and they might resort to making you feel guilty when your other relationships demand your attention too. This behavior is unhealthy because by isolating you from your other relationships, they are tethering you tightly to them. Your other relationships are like a support system, and you need them to have a happy, fulfilled, and balanced life. No one can survive with just one relationship alone. Whether your partner does it on purpose or unknowingly, isolation sews seeds of self-doubt. Healthy love is independent, where the people involved in that relationship enjoy spending time together, but still stay connected to the activities and the people they cared about *before*. Maintaining your independence is one of the primary indicators of a healthy relationship.

- **One Person In the Relationship Is Extremely Jealous** - In a codependent relationship, that extreme jealousy could manifest into unhealthy behavior patterns. The jealous person could become overly emotional, lash out, become unpredictable, and in even more extreme cases, resort to violence or aggression. This indicator tends to manifest in romantic relationships more so than anything else. Your insecure, possibly codependent partner might want to know where you are and who you're with at all times because they have come to rely on you so much they can't bear the thought of losing you. The notion of them not being able to live without you might sound romantic, but nothing could be further from the truth. You see, extreme jealousy brings with it mistrust and possessiveness too, and they could refuse to listen to reason when their emotions get in the way of logical thinking. While jealousy is a part of any normal human relationship, the indicative difference here is extreme jealousy. Extreme jealousy can be threatening, angry, and desperate, none of which should exist in a healthy relationship dynamic.

- **Too Many Highs and Lows** - Frequent breakups and then makeups, highs, lows, ups, and downs that are so frequent they have become emotionally draining and exhausting. That is an indicator you're in an unhealthy relationship. The danger of this emotional roller coaster is that words can be said in anger, hurt, and frustration, and these are words that hurt. Words that can leave a scar that you might never recover from. These words are then quickly followed by an emotional and teary apology, promising never to do that again, yet the same thing happens the next time an emotional roller coaster episode happens again. When you're in a codependent relationship for too long, you're in danger of becoming so accustomed to this behavior that you no longer realize how dangerous and unhealthy the relationship has become.

Once you understand the signs of unhealthy love, it can help you assess nearly every relationship in your life. Once you have opened your eyes to the signs, you might understand for the first time in your life why you feel disappointed by friendship, or why you might feel betrayed by a family member. Maybe you start to understand why an encounter with certain people in your life could leave you feeling discouraged, anxious, or unhappy. You might even start to realize if you have been guilty of displaying signs of being the codependent one in your relationships without realizing it. Understanding is the very first step toward improving and ultimately curing yourself of the codependent relationships in your life once and for all. Understanding these signs will also help you avoid the rabbit hole that leads to unhealthy love, and this is going to improve every relationship you have in your life.

A relationship *should never* define your value, or be a source of your emotional health and happiness.

CHAPTER 2

Why Codependent Relationships Are Never Healthy

The path to recovery is not always an easy one, especially for unhealthy relationships. It's going to make you flinch and cringe several times along the way because part of the recovery process involves opening your eyes to the truth. The truth is not always going to be pretty.

The Mind and It's Duality

The mind is a powerful thing. It lives in a dual world, the conscious and the subconscious/unconscious. Certain situations and circumstances, like codependency, live in the subconscious mind. The subconscious mind is where we store all the habits and ways of operating that we don't give much thought to. The functions that happen daily on autopilot are happening from the subconscious mind. The subconscious mind is the one responsible for making us reactive. By nature, we are reactive. We react to the people around us, we react to what we see before us, and we react to everything that is happening in our lives. The subconscious mind also happens to be responsible for a lot of the denial we live in.

When it comes to codependency, the subconscious mind is absolutely in denial. The first sign that codependency is a situation where denial plays a heavy hand is when we *deny ourselves*. We forget that we are individuals. We have our own needs, wants, desires, dreams, ambitions, and more. We have our own way of doing things, but we don't give much thought to that when we find ourselves in a codependent relationship. We brush it off and convince ourselves that the other person's needs matter more than ours do. Living in this form of denial causes the codependent one to seek external validation, driven by a strong desire to please others. The codependent person prefers to focus all of their time, energy, and attention on that one primary person they have come to rely so heavily upon. They would quite literally do anything to keep the relationship from falling apart.

Now, you might be wondering what is the harm if I want to make someone I love or care about happy? What is wrong with that? Why does this create such a messy situation? The answer to those questions is because you end up being nothing more than an extension of someone else. When you're so busy focusing on other people, you are not checking in with *yourself*. You are not focusing on your own reality and eventually, you will lose yourself along the way. That is one of the reasons why you're holding on so tightly to a relationship that is unhealthy for you. You become so afraid of losing this relationship because, in your subconscious mind, you're afraid you don't know who you would be without this person in your life.

Codependency Is Living In A World of Denial

Besides leading to your subconscious mind suppressing all the parts of yourself and your relationship that you are afraid to confront, codependency also to denial that your relationship might be abusive. Perhaps not physically abusive, but mentally and emotionally. If you're struggling with low self-esteem, came from an erratic, abusive, or unpredictable childhood or home life growing up, there is a tendency to be in denial of others. For example, if you grew up with parents who might have habitually neglected you or never gave you the support that you needed. Since these are your parents, people whom you love and the very same people you believe should love you too, you condition yourself to be in denial.

As you move forward and form other relationships in your life, that initial relationship denial never goes away. Not only will you be in denial that your relationship might be abusive in some way, but you will also be in denial about the person you're *in love with*. If they are not good people, you will find a way to ignore or deny it and stay in the relationship longer than you should. You make excuses for them, tell yourself what you need to believe that this is real love, you discount their behavior, and you choose to sweep the unhealthy parts of the relationship under the rug rather than confront the truth. If you were to confront them about it, you're likely to believe any story they tell you because you want to believe it. Once again, that is just another example of how you would do anything to hold onto a relationship, even if deep down, you know that you shouldn't.

Living in denial is never a good thing. You don't know how to set boundaries, you don't know how to function should you lose the person you're depending on, and you allow yourself to believe that no matter what kind of life you have with this person, it is still better to be with them than to be without them. What is worse is that this kind of denial is going to plummet your self-esteem and self-worth, eroding it slowly over time until you don't recognize the person that you are anymore. If at some point in the future the relationship does come to an end, you're at a loss. You don't know who you are or what your purpose is anymore.

When you're a codependent person, you tend to live in denial of your own experiences and instincts too. This is no way to live your life because when you start living for the sake of other people, that's not a life that is going to make you happy. You start doing things because you think it's going to make the other person happy instead of thinking about what makes *you* happy. It is important to realize that when you are codependent, you're completely checked out from your internal experiences. You're not living mindfully, and you're not paying attention to your emotions and your needs. This is causing you a great deal of unhappiness, but you're denying this too. To aid in the recovery process, it is important to realize how deeply affected by denial you are and why codependent relationships are so unhealthy for this very reason.

You Lose Your Sense of Value

Many people out there in codependent relationships believe that their value is directly proportional to how much they can do for others or how they treat other people. You believe that if you go out of your way to do things for them, you're more valuable to the relationship somehow. But this kind of thinking is *flawed.* Yes, it is good to treat other people with respect. Yes, it is okay to do things for the people you love. Yes, it is okay to be nice to others. *But your value is not directly reflected in those factors.* Your value and sense of self-worth is something that comes from within.

Self-love is an important aspect of your overall wellbeing. It affects the decisions that you make, how you see yourself, and the relationships you have with others.

Self-love can only exist when you value yourself, and this is something that cannot happen when you continue to live your life based on other people. Depending on your circumstances or the way that you grew up, valuing and loving yourself can be extremely difficult for some people. This is how you end up in codependent relationships. If you suspect that a lack of self-love and not valuing yourself enough could be one of the contributing factors behind your codependent tendencies, these are some signs you can watch out for:

- **You're Not Confident** - This sign is by far the most obvious indicator that you don't value and love yourself enough. If you realize that you have a history of bouncing from one unhappy relationship to the next, this is the reason. Since you're not confident, you never speak up and voice your opinions in the relationship. You go with the flow of what other people want because it's easier to make them happy rather than say what you would like to do instead.

- **You Tend to Hide Who You Truly Are from Others** - You're afraid that if people saw or got to know the real you, they wouldn't love you for who you are. You feel like you have to be a chameleon, changing your personality to fit the person or group of people you are with at the time. You put on a proverbial mask to hide certain parts of your personality from others, especially the one that you have become so heavily dependent on. All of this is rooted in the fear and belief that people will leave you once they see who you truly were. This kind of thinking can only exist when you don't love or value yourself enough. You're worried about being judged or that you're not worthy enough, in a way, as you hide and pretend to be someone that you are not, hoping to hold on to those relationships for as long as you can. You try to change your behavior based on what the other person needs, even if it makes you unhappy to do it.

- **You Tend to Overanalyze Your Own Behavior -** Being codependent will make you overanalyze your own behavior. A lot. Once again, this is because of that deep-seated, subconscious fear you have of losing your relationships. You're paranoid and overthink almost everything you do because you are desperate to hang on to your relationships. When you don't love and value yourself enough, your brain has a tendency to focus and magnify all the perceived flaws in your personality.

- **You Need Affirmation and Attention -** While it is nice to hear praise and recognition from others once in a while, a codependent person that lacks self-love is going to need excessive amounts of attention and affirmation. They need constant reassurance from the other person that they are doing okay. They need attention from their primary dependent and become distressed when they don't get it. In the long run, this can put a tremendous strain on the relationship, emotionally taxing you and the people around you. No one can give you the attention you need twenty-four hours a day, seven days a week. Everyone has their own life to live, and this is yet another example of why being codependent on others for love and affirmation is an unhealthy habit to carry.

- **You're Terrified of Being Judged** - You're terrified of being judged by others, even more so by the person you're in a codependent relationship with. You love and care about each other, yet at the same time, you're afraid that they are going to judge you if you do anything that makes them upset or unhappy. This is responsible for a lot of the people-pleasing tendencies you exhibit when you're in a codependent relationship.

- **You Struggle With the Idea of Self-Care** - You have a hard time believing that you deserve to treat yourself right. The idea of taking some time off to nurture your mind, body, and soul is something you cannot fathom without being riddled with guilt. You would rather neglect to build your own happiness in favor of focusing on your partner's needs (if you are in a romantic relationship).

- **You Feel Inferior** - You have put the person you're dependent on so high up on a pedestal that you feel inferior to them. You are convinced that they are better than you in every way, and therefore, you are the unworthy and inferior one in the relationship. You're judging yourself harshly all the time and beat yourself up over the simplest mistakes. You diminish your accomplishments and the only thing you can focus on are your failures and shortcomings, all of which contribute to the fear that you are going to lose the relationship you've come to depend on.

When you don't value and love yourself enough, it can create an unhealthy relationship dynamic. In any kind of relationship, both people involved need to consider themselves equal partners. If one always fears inferior to the other, it is going to put a strain on that relationship, and it doesn't matter if it is a romantic relationship, friendship, or the bonds you have with your family. Without self-love, you will always be settling for less than you deserve, making it impossible to find lasting happiness. Being codependent will make you fail to realize that a relationship should never be responsible for your happiness. That it should never be the sole reason for your happiness. Happiness, like self-love and valuing yourself, is something that must come from within. You, and you alone, are responsible for your own happiness.

Love Is Never Unhealthy

Love is an instinctive emotion. It is an emotion that feels *good*. It is an emotion that envelops you with warmth and happiness. Love, when it is *real* love in its purest form, is happiness. Yet, a lot of people struggle to understand this emotion because they don't realize that love should never be unhealthy. When it's love, you're never going to be left feeling confused, unsure of where you stand, or even what's going on. You feel comfortable, and you'll never have to feel like you need to be on your guard. There won't be this nagging feeling in your gut, telling you that something may not be quite right. But like all emotions, even true love can become toxic when we continue to ignore the warning signs. In a codependent relationship, these unhealthy signs that indicate the love that is present might not be real or healthy can be blurred or ignored completely.

- **Real Love Is Stable** - At the start of any new relationship, everything always feels new and incredible. The rush of emotions, the high intensity of affections, the euphoria that you feel when you're together is what keeps us addicted to wanting to feel that way. When the relationship is healthy and not codependent, these emotions will stabilize over time. That is not the case with unhealthy, codependent love. The emotions will always feel like a roller coaster, highs, and lows, exhausting and draining. When your relationship begins to feel like too much hard work, too intense, and smothering rather than euphoric, you know that this love has become unhealthy.

- **Real Love Never Feels the Need to Hide Anything** - The minute you feel like you can't be yourself, that you must keep parts of your personality hidden from your partner because they wouldn't approve, that is not what love is anymore. That's codependency. Love means being completely comfortable to have even difficult conversations with your partner and feel assured that they're going to love and support your decisions if it's going to be for the best. If you have to pretend, tell little white lies and keep secrets just to avoid upsetting your partner, that's no longer a sign of a healthy relationship.

- **Real Love Has A Sense of Independence** - Yes, you do miss the one you love when they are not around, but it doesn't feel like your world is about to collapse when you have to be on your own. You can still function independently, and you don't feel the need to keep asking their opinion to go after your own pursuits.

- **Real Love Has No Problem with Disagreements** - When the love is real and not codependent, you don't fear disagreements. In fact, even when you're disagreeing, a loving relationship that is healthy allows you to have these disagreements and arguments while still maintaining mutual respect for each other. Love will never make you feel guilty either for having to say no when you want to. Partners, friends, or family members who love each other will never judge, ridicule, make one person feel bad over for their opinions or actions, and they'll never blame each other for all the problems that happen while assuming no responsibility on their part.

- **Real Love Will Never Feel Like You Are Forced to Do Anything** - Love never forces one person to do something they don't want to do. Love will never try to control your actions and only force you to behave in a certain way. With love, you're free to be yourself and be happy about it, knowing that your partner loves you just the way you are. If you constantly have to set aside your own needs and desires just to accommodate your partner, you might be in a manipulative relationship. If they constantly make you feel like the worst person in the world when you have to turn down their requests, they're manipulating you. If they give you an ultimatum that forces you to action, that is not what love is either.

All relationships will have their ups and downs, but when the love is real, there will always be one element that is present despite the disagreements. *Happiness.* Despite the ups and downs that you experience in a relationship, a healthy relationship is still one that is going to be happy. Even during the hard times, love still makes you feel happy because you can find comfort and support in each other. It infuses you with positive feelings. A codependent and unhealthy relationship is the opposite. It is hard to feel happy in a relationship if your happiness revolves around other people. Healthy love is always selfless and giving. To put it simply, a codependent relationship is toxic.

Toxic Relationships Will Never Be Good for You

No matter how much you try to justify it or the number of excuses you make for yours or their behavior, a codependent relationship will never be good for you. If there is one thing you can be sure of, it is that codependent relationships are toxic in their own way, and toxic relationships will never have a happy ending. It may be "happy" for a little while, but if it isn't going to last, the happiness was never real, to begin with. You start to get comfortable with it and make excuses for being in that toxic relationship because it feels better than having to deal with the pain of letting go of the person that you love. If you feel like you constantly have to work overtime to hold on to that sense of happiness, it was never yours to start with. A codependent relationship is toxic, and it will leave its impact on you in one way or another.

- **A Toxic Relationship Will Make You More Guarded** - It will be difficult to trust anybody. Codependency results in two individuals placing an excessive amount of emotional and even psychological reliance on the other. The intensity of this relationship would differ depending on the couple, but at the end of that relationship, it will feel like a struggle to trust anyone. Your experience with this kind of toxic relationship may make you more suspicious of others. You find yourself always wondering what their true intentions are of whether they are sincere when they tell you that they care about you. When you lose yourself in a toxic relationship, your judgment becomes clouded and it is harder to see what is best for yourself anymore. The irony is, you end up getting even more hurt because you find it difficult to trust anybody.

- **Codependency Is A Breeding Ground of Negativity** - Being one form of a toxic relationship, codependency becomes a breeding ground for negativity. When you are unhappy deep inside, you're opening the door for a lot of unhealthy, unhappy thoughts to come creeping in bit by bit. Your life is filled with worry and fear. You lose touch with your own goals, passions, desires, ambitions, and purpose. You change your opinions for the sake of keeping the peace. Their problems begin to bother you as if it were your own problems. A codependent relationship is toxic because it lacks emotional support or expression of approval. They are unhealthy, imbalanced, and lack moral, positive, or even ethical principles. Not only that, but they are unpleasant to be around. Being happy when you're in a toxic relationship is impossible, no matter how hard you try to convince yourself otherwise. Nothing is a bigger energy drainer than spending all of your efforts making sure the other person is happy but not receiving the same kind of support in return.

- **Codependency Makes You Pessimistic** - Being in a toxic relationship can drastically alter your views on life. This can happen even if the relationship has ended for a while now. You're emotionally exhausted from being so pessimistic all the time, but you don't know how to stop feeling and thinking this way. Being around somebody who is toxic for too long will make you feel bad about yourself, insecure, drained, stressed, pressured, and even emotionally scarred. If you find yourself doing things or exhibiting patterns of behavior that are out of character whenever you're around a codependent person, it is a sure sign that they have more power in your life than they should. You know that you're giving them the power whenever you let their behavior negatively influence your own behavior. You let your emotions get the better of you, and each time you do something that is not who you usually are, you're letting the codependent toxic person influence you more than you should.

- **A Codependent Relationship Will Wear Down Your Self-Image** - Another reason why such a relationship is toxic is that it will affect your self-image eventually. When you spend all that time and energy focused on someone else instead of yourself, it's hard not to feel bad about yourself.

- **A Toxic and Codependent Relationship Will Hinder Your Personal Growth** - This is another side effect of not focusing on yourself and your own needs enough. All your time and energy is being channeled toward someone else that you don't have time to work on your personal growth anymore. Many codependent people find themselves stuck in one place, watching everyone else around them move forward with their lives. They feel sad, jealous, envious, miserable, and unhappy, wondering why their life feels stagnant and why it is so difficult for them to achieve their dreams while other people make it look effortless. When you have a hard time answering questions about who you are and what matters to you, it is time to admit that your relationship is toxic. It doesn't matter how much you want to hold on to that relationship, it is never going to be good for you if it hinders your personal growth.

CHAPTER 3

Eleven Key Symptoms To Look For And How To Recover

Chapter 3:

If you're worried that codependence might be something that is troubling your relationship, there is a way to tell if your suspicions might be true. Codependency is a struggle for many, and one of the aspects that a lot of people struggle with is identifying the signs. It can be a real problem, especially when it gets in the way of you having healthy, happy relationships. The kind of relationships that you deserve. The kind of relationship you always dreamed of having, not only with your significant other but with every person in your life. No matter how independent or strong we are, we cannot run away from the fact that at the end of the day, we're only human. As humans, we are all driven by one basic instinct. *The need to connect to others.*

What Are the Eleven Key Signs?

Do you believe that you might have a codependency problem? Is your significant other a codependent person? The boundary between healthy and unhealthy dependence is when you (or someone that you have a relationship with) has come to depend on another in such an extreme way they cannot function without them. If you, or someone that you know, simply refuse to do *anything* without the person you suspect they are dependent on, your suspicions might be right after all. Unhealthy codependency boils down to the *need to be needed*. You either *want* to be needed by another, or someone else *needs* you in nearly every aspect of their lives they can no longer function well independently.

You can't shake this nagging feeling that you might be overly reliant on your partners, friends, or family. That your emotional needs go beyond what might be normal. Perhaps you have been called "needy" or "clingy" in the past. Like all problems, codependency does display some subtle warning signs, and these are the eleven signs to start paying attention to if your gut is telling you that you might have a codependent problem:

- **Key Sign #1: You Feel Responsible for Other People's Problems** - Every adult should be able to solve and figure out their own problems. That is part of what it means to be an adult. However, when it comes to a point where you feel responsible for solving other people's problems, you might have a codependency problem. You feel a strong urge or desire to fix other people's problems, even if it causes you a great deal of stress. You believe that if you can't help them fix their problems, they are going to leave you or abandon this relationship. You go out of your way at times to help them fix a problem, even if they tell you that they can handle it. At times, you feel upset if someone you care about tells you they can handle their problems on their own and they don't need your help right now. That urge you feel to be needed by them starts triggering all sorts of anxious thoughts in your mind, causing immense stress and fear that you're no longer valuable or needed in the relationship anymore. Codependent people are likely to believe that if they cannot help the people in their lives, then nobody is going to want to have them around. It is not your responsibility to fix other people's problems, but the codependent person in you won't let you take a step back and relax.

- **Key Sign #2: You Feel the Need to Be In Control** - This need is not something that crops up once in a while. This is an ongoing need *all the time.* When you feel like you're not in control, your anxiety gets triggered. You feel such a strong desire and need to be in control that you try to avoid conflict and upset at any cost. Every little detail must be planned out and carried out *exactly* the way you want it too. Perhaps you might have been accused of being uptight or anal at some point. You do things you don't want to do, say things you don't want to say, act in ways you might not feel comfortable with, and you do all of this to gain some sense of control. The thought of not having any control brings up severe panic in you because it feels like everything is spinning out of control. Depending on how extreme your circumstances are, a lack of control could, at times, trigger a panic attack. All of this is also driven by the fear that if you're not fulfilling a purpose in the relationship, then you are not needed.

- **Key Sign #3: It Is Nearly Impossible For You to Say No -** You always end up giving *too much* because you struggle with the idea of saying no. The very thought of having to say no triggers your fears about being left or abandoned, and you feel so terrified over the thought of losing the relationship you end up saying yes even when you wanted to say no. You say yes when you're too tired, you say yes when you feel stressed, you say yes when you're far too busy dealing with everything that is on your plate as it is, and you keep saying yes until you're burned out and can't go on anymore. You end up giving more in the relationship compared to the other person. Your fear has convinced you that the survival of your relationship depends on your ability to say yes to every request that is asked of you. It feels like you are responsible for keeping the relationship together, and this is a heavy burden that weighs on your shoulders. You feel stressed about it, but you don't want to say anything and risk jeopardizing the relationship.

- **Key Sign #4: You Feel Upset When It Seems Like Your Efforts Are Not Being Recognized -** When it feels like people are not praising or recognizing all the hard work you are putting into the relationship, you sometimes feel upset, hurt, jealous, angry, bitter, or resentful. You are doing a lot in the relationship, like the point above mentions, and because you're doing a lot, there will be a little resentment or frustration when you feel like you are not getting the recognition you deserve. The problem is that no one else might have asked you to do all this extra work. It is driven by your internal need to feel important and valuable in the relationship. But, some part of you is still going to be upset about the fact that your efforts might not be recognized the way that you hoped.

- **Key Sign #5: You Find It Very Difficult to Trust Yourself** - You have a hard time trusting yourself, and this explains why you struggle to make decisions without the approval of others. If you have that primary person in the relationship that you have formed an attachment to, you struggle to do anything without their approval. If they don't like it, you're not going to do it (even though you want to). You're terrified of making a mistake should you act on your own because you're afraid that mistake is going to cost you your relationship. You carry a lot of pressure with you, constantly worried about people giving up on you if you make a mistake. You live each day in fear that one mistake is going to cause your relationship to unravel, and this makes you second guess yourself when you need to make a decision or take some form of action. You feel the pressure to do everything perfectly, meet everyone's needs, be what you think other people expect you to be, and once more, you feel this heavy burden on your shoulders to get it right all the time. It is exhausting.

- **Key Sign #6: You Attach Your Value to How Much You Can "Save" or "Fix" People** - It's not enough for you to be yourself in the relationship and enjoy it as it is. Your codependent tendencies have convinced you that your value is based on how much you're able to contribute to the relationship by "fixing" or "saving" other people. You believe it is your responsibility in some way to get them through their problems, despite the fact that they are perfectly capable of doing it on their own. This explains why, for example, you might overlook your partner's gambling problem and cover up for them instead of getting them the help that they need. You believe that it is your job to fix everything around them and help them deal with your stuff to show that you care about the relationship. You might even find yourself purposely looking for something to be fixed, and if there is nothing, you're restless and uneasy. You don't wait for them to ask for you for help, you do it because you're codependent.

- **Key Sign #7: You Struggle With Trying to Identify Your Own Feelings** - You have a hard time identifying with the way that you feel because you're constantly thinking about other people. You're so busy trying to meet other people's needs that you don't know what your own needs are anymore. You don't even know how to feel when something happens in the relationship that relates to you. Instead of trying to process your emotions, you start scrambling and trying to find a way to turn the focus back to the other person. You have become so used to being there and doing things for other people that you're *afraid* to think about your own feelings because you have lost sight of who you are. You don't know what is important to you anymore, and this is one of the many reasons why codependency is only going to make you unhappy, no matter how much you try to convince yourself otherwise.

- **Key Sign #8: You Would Do Anything to Hold On To That Relationship** - You would do anything, even if it was destructive or unsafe. Driven by your desire to hold on to the relationship at any cost, there might be times when you would be willing to put yourself at risk if it means you're not going to lose the relationship. You compromise too much. You look the other way more often than you should. You ignore the red flags and the warning signs by convincing yourself that it is no big deal. You tell yourself that the relationship is worth risking it all for, even when deep down, you know that it is killing you to do it. When we're in an unhealthy relationship, part of us knows it. Our subconscious mind knows it. Our gut knows it. Yet, we choose to ignore it because we would rather put up with anything if it means we don't have to be alone. That is what unhealthy codependency would make you do, and this is very risky as it could put you in danger of doing some pretty uncompromising things for the sake of holding onto something that you should be letting go of.

- **Key Sign #9: You Feel Guilty Making It About You** - You never want to speak up in the relationship because you feel guilty. You feel like if you do speak up and say what is on your mind, you're going to be perceived as selfish. You're afraid that people are going to get fed up with you if you keep voicing your needs and ditch the relationship, leaving you all alone yet again. You're willing to put your own health and safety at risk if it means the people in your life are going to love you a little bit more. Your codependent self might convince you that any risk is worth taking if it means other people realize that they *need* you around.

- **Key Sign #10: You Tend to Choose Partners Who Are In Need** - Because you are driven by your desire to feel needed and to fix others, you might subconsciously be choosing "problematic" partners without even knowing it. You choose partners who have problems that need to be fixed, partners who are in crisis or get into relationships with people who have issues because you think you can help to make them better. You could find yourself in a lot of relationships with people who have mental health issues, addiction issues, or any other problems where you see yourself being needed. In other words, you are getting into a lot of unhealthy relationships for all the wrong reasons. You *think* you can make it better when really all you are doing is creating more problems for yourself.

- **Key Sign #11: You Need to Be Reassured -** When you don't get the reassurance that you need, you feel anxious and stressed like you are not doing enough to keep the other person happy. You're either asking the other person to tell you that you have done a good job, or you are hoping that they will each time you go the extra mile. You don't realize that you're subconsciously doing all these extra things for the relationship because you are hoping to get verbal approval from the other person.

A common theme you will notice among all these indicators is fear. You're primarily driven by the fear of either losing the relationship or the fear of being alone. The one thing you can be sure of is that codependency is going to put a lot of strain on your relationship, for both you and the people involved. Your codependent tendencies are damaging to both you and the relationship because it is simply not realistic to fix problems all the time. It is not possible to keep the relationship happy all the time. Relationships go through ups and downs, that is how it is supposed to be. Setting unreasonable expectations is only setting yourself up for inevitable disappointment. When you tie your self-worth and your value to your ability to fix other people's problems all the time, you are only setting yourself up for failure and unhappiness.

You Need to Learn to Say "No"

For many people, saying no is *very, very difficult.* Saying "no" doesn't feel great. In fact, it makes you feel like an awful person, having to say no to someone in need, especially if it is someone you love and care about. Nobody wants to feel like the bad guy. When you have codependency issues, saying no is going to feel like an impossible thing to do. You know you're tired. You know you're reaching your limit. You know you're getting exhausted. You know that your stress levels seem to be climbing higher every day. But the codependent part of you continues to ignore the small murmurs that are tugging at your sleeve, telling you to say "no" because you're afraid of the consequences that might follow. Saying no is one of the hardest things to do for a codependent, yet it is something you *must* learn how to do if you hope to cure yourself of this unhealthy attachment that you have.

You *need to* put a stop to your fear of saying no. Letting go of this fear is the only way to begin work on your recovery process. You cannot cure yourself of codependency if you keep worrying that people are going to leave you if you say no to them. Yes, it is not a bad thing to want to make the people you love happy, and no one is saying that it is. When you care about the person, naturally you want to do what you can to keep them happy. But there is a point when this desire to keep the people in your life happy becomes unhealthy, and that point is when you start neglecting yourself. Evidence that you're starting to neglect your needs in favor of theirs is when you agree to something, do it reluctantly, but think to yourself "I cannot refuse" because you don't want to upset them or let them down. If you had to say "no," you feel guilty for days on end, maybe even weeks, and each time you see them, that guilt is fresh in your mind. You believe you're hurting them when you say "no," and this stops you from doing it, even when you know that you should.

Saying no does not make you a bad person. Being afraid of rejection by your peers and loved ones is not uncommon. If you fear being rejected, you are not alone. Nobody wants to feel like they are not wanted, we all have an innate desire to be accepted. Some may even find themselves doing things in their relationships that are not necessarily who they are as a person simply because they worry about being rejected if they don't. The people you genuinely love and care about you will never leave you because you say no to them once in a while. Saying no is something every healthy relationship experiences once in a while. If you keep saying yes all the time, somebody is going to feel unhappy. Most of the time, the unhappy one is going to be you if you're the codependent one. Not all relationships are going to be good for you. Some relationships can be so disruptive they strip you of your happiness and your focus. When you're miserable, it becomes difficult to concentrate on anything, let alone trying to focus on what you need to be happy. This is even more challenging if you happen to get into a relationship where the other person is equally as codependent as you are.

You Are Not the Bad Guy for Saying No

As hard as it is to say no, you must learn how to do it. If you don't, you're going to keep feeling overwhelmed, frustrated, stressed out, and all the other emotions that are only going to make you unhappy. Your feelings and your emotions matter just as much as anyone else. Your needs and desires deserve to be understood too. Your feelings and emotions matter. We all want to love and be loved in return, but it's hard to feel loved when you constantly feel like you're being misunderstood by the people you want desperately to connect with. You matter, and this is something you might have to frequently remind yourself of until the message sticks in your mind. For healthy relationships to exist, limits need to be in place. It sets the standard from the beginning for mutual respect from all parties involved, and this enables a happier co-existence all around. The happier you are with the relationships in your life, the more you will flourish as a person.

You are responsible for the happiness that you experience in your relationship, and to experience this happiness, you need to be responsible for what you say yes and no too. A codependent person can only start breaking out of this habit by overcoming the fear of saying no, and this is how you do it while feeling as little guilt as possible:

- **Baby Steps and Starting Small** - You will never be able to please everyone, no matter who they are. It's hard to go cold turkey and flat out say "no" right away to everyone, and if you do feel this way, start small and work your way up from there. No one should pressure you into deciding or taking an action you're not comfortable with, and if they love you, they will be okay with it. It is okay to make an active choice to work on your own happiness first, and once you've created that better life for yourself, those positive choices will carry over to the environment around you, including the people that you love. You can make your own decisions, your own choices, and if you choose to say no, go right ahead. Practice with the small "no's" first. For example, if you don't feel like going to a party but you feel bad about it, say you'll be there but you're coming a little later so you don't have to stay through the entire thing. Compromise. It's about finding balance and accepting the fact that just because you can't please everyone, it doesn't make you a horrible person.

- **Listen to Your Heart** - If your mind, body, and every fiber of your being is telling you to say no, then it is time that you listened to it. Your feelings and your emotions matter just as much as anyone else. If something doesn't feel quite right, you don't have to go through with it, no matter what other people may try to convince you of. Respect your emotions enough to stand firm on your boundaries and say no with anything you're not happy to agree with. Make yourself happy first before working on making someone else happy. You can't spend the rest of your life worried about making mistakes. This is a message you need to yourself as many times as needed until it sticks in your mind. No matter how much you love them or care about them, you cannot spend the rest of your life worrying about what is going to happen if you say no to them.

- **If It's Not A Resounding Yes, Then It's A No** - This is the easiest way to help you make a decision. You know the difference when you want to say yes to something. Think about the times where you've had a request and immediately you were thrilled to say yes without even thinking about it. A resounding yes that you were thrilled to agree to. That is the kind of feeling you want to emulate for every request. If it is not a resounding yes, then it is going to be a no.

The desire to want to help the people in your life is not a bad thing. But you have to remember that you only have twenty-four hours in a day. There is only so much you can do without stretching yourself too thin. It is not worth it to keep pushing yourself because when you are tired and stressed out, you can't give the very best parts of yourself to the relationship anyway. Learn to say no, it is going to make a big difference in the way that you interact with others. Just remember that the ones who truly love you are never going to leave because you said no once in a while.

CHAPTER 4

Why Narcissistic Partners Seek To Manipulate You

To say that being in a relationship with someone who is narcissistic is challenging would be an understatement. A narcissist is not just someone who thinks they are the best thing to walk the earth. There is a lot more to the narcissist than most people realize. Unless you're in a relationship with one, or you have experience being with a narcissist in the past, you wouldn't know what it is truly like being around these manipulative, selfish, and conceited personalities. For a regular person, dating a narcissist on its own is challenging. For someone who is codependent, the struggles are even harder.

Who Is A Narcissist Anyway?

A narcissist is someone who projects an air of self-importance. They project a false version of themselves to avoid dealing with who they truly are. The more severe forms of narcissism are classified under the DSM-5 as *Narcissistic Personality Disorder*. The DSM-5 is the Diagnostic and Statistical Manual of Mental Disorders, and it classifies those diagnosed with *Narcissistic Personality Disorder* as someone who expects to be recognized as superior, even if they are not that extraordinary, to begin with. Those with *Narcissistic Personality Disorder* require excessive amounts of admiration.

They also have a very strong sense of entitlement, and this means they will not have any problems taking advantage of others in the pursuit of their own self-interest. If it means they get what they want, they will be willing to step on your toes and stab you in the back. They don't care about anyone else's happiness as much as they care about their own. This includes people they supposedly claim to love. The truth is, a narcissist will love themselves *first* before they love anyone else. They have exaggerated levels of self-esteem. They believe they are the picture of perfection and to themselves, they are infallible. Depending on the individual in question, the strength of the narcissistic tendencies would vary in strength, with some people having a stronger disposition towards this personality than others. Narcissism is associated with grandiosity, a distinct lack of empathy, egotism, and pride.

What Does This Mean If I'm In A Relationship With A Narcissist?

Being in a relationship with a narcissist is both painful and traumatizing, especially if you're someone who is codependent. Your partner could be causing you a lot of pain, hurt, and grief, yet you can't bring yourself to leave them because you're so dependent on them. This begs the question of why anyone would enter into a relationship with a narcissist in the first place. The answer is because they can be *very* charismatic. The charm you into falling in love with them, and they are experts at making you believe you are the most special person in the world to them. They *want* you to care about them because they know this means you will give them the attention that they crave. To get what they want, a narcissist will pretend to care about you too, something that is easy enough to achieve during the courtship stage of the relationship. Everyone is always on their best behavior early on as each partner tries to impress the other.

A narcissist will shower their prospective partner with so much love and affection that they can't think clearly. They'll whisper sweet nothings to you and promise you everything that you want to hear. Everything that you have been longing to hear for so long. They'll promise you the sky and the moon, and they will make you believe that you have finally found the one who is perfect for you. They'll sweep you off your feet and make you fall head over heels in love with them, and you won't realize their true colors until it is too late. Once they've got you hooked if you're a codependent person, that's all they need. The minute you stop giving them what they want, however, their charm is going to disappear faster than you can snap your fingers together.

No doubt about it, the narcissist is manipulative and dangerous. They have no intention of doing any of the things they promised you they would do. They will never respect your boundaries either since they believe they are entitled to do anything and everything that they want. They are preoccupied with nothing but their own self-interests, and your boundaries go against their self-interest. Therefore, they'll seek to push you to your limits, even more so if they know you are someone who is codependent. They'll be delighted to find out that you can't bear the thought of losing them since this works in their favor tremendously.

The Signs You're Dating A Narcissist

Here are the signs you could be dating a narcissist that is taking advantage of your codependent nature:

- **It's All About Them** - They only want to talk about themselves all the time. It is always about *their* needs, *their* wants, and they will always find a way to make themselves the subject of every conversation. Every story and every reference will always lead back to them, and when they know you're codependent, willing to do whatever it takes to make them happy, you can be sure they are going to milk it for everything that it is worth. They want to be the center of attention all the time because they like it that way. If they are not in the spotlight, they will find a way to be. Some narcissistic partners might even like to hear *you talk about them.* They have no qualms about asking you self-centered questions like, *"What do you like most about me?".* While it is normal to ask these kinds of questions once in a while, especially when you may be genuinely curious about how your partner feels about you, a narcissist likes to ask these conceited questions on a regular basis.

- **They Use Language That Is Exaggerated** - It is not only the subject of the conversation that comes off as self-centered. A narcissist tends to use the same kind of arrogance and self-important language when they talk about themselves. A narcissist has a way of portraying themselves in a way that makes them appear wonderful in every story. In some stories, they will depict themselves as the "hero" who saves the day. For example, a regular person who finds a wallet on the street would probably tell the story as it is. They would then say they were relieved to find the wallet's owner, or say that they turned the wallet over to the proper authorities to deal with it. A narcissist, however, will spin the story in an exaggerated fashion because they crave the admiration of others. A narcissist would exaggerate almost every detail to spice up the story if it means they can squeeze as much admiration and awe out of you as possible.

- **They Lack Flexible Empathy** - Your narcissistic partner could have unreasonably high expectations of you. Many narcissistic partners tend to be very unforgiving because they lack the ability to be flexible. For example, if you were running late and met them ten minutes later than what you promised, they might yell at you and make a big deal out of it the same way they would if you had crashed their car. They want you to be perfect and they expect you to live up to their expectations. Since the narcissist genuinely believes the world revolves around them, it is all about *you* bending over backward to meet their demands and expectations. The moment you fail or disappoint them in any way, they are going to lash out at you.

- **They Never Follow Through On What They Say** - A narcissist is all talk and no action. They are good at talking a big game, but when it comes time to back up their words, they consistently fall short. If your partner never follows through on what they promise, then you are probably dating a narcissist. If your codependent tendencies mean that you are always the one to pick up the slack, then you can be sure that they are *never* going to follow through because they know that you will do it. They will always tell you and make it seem like they have everything under control, but they rarely ever do. The lack of consistency should be a huge red flag for you. If you cannot depend on your partner to have your back when you need it most because they never follow through, the relationship is doomed to struggle. In any relationship, you should always be able to count on your partner to have your back. A relationship is a teamwork, and if one member of the team falls short, that team is going to struggle every step of the way.

- **They Don't Like Being Told What to Do -** To them, they should be the ones *telling you* what to do, not the other way around. The minute you try and tell them what to do, they could become angry or defensive, making all sorts of excuses and trying to turn the tables back on you. They will make it seem like you are the one in the wrong for even suggesting it. They can't stand the idea of being told what to do, and they will try to exert their "power" to prove a point that no one can tell them what to do. Although they don't like being told what to do, they have no problems trying to *control you.* They don't mind telling you what they think you should do. The narcissist will try to control everything that you do, say, and even think. If you're in a relationship with them, they will try to control your conversation, what you wear, what you eat, where you go, who you talk to, even the things you're allowed to buy. The conversation will always seem to revolve around them and their needs, and even if you were to mention or try and raise an issue that concerns you, they'll be quick to dismiss it and spin the conversation right back around to them. To make matters worse, they will attempt to make you feel bad for raising your concerns while they were in the middle of talking about themselves.

- **They Need to Be Validated** - A narcissist believes that nothing is worth doing unless there are other people around to witness it and praise them for it. Do you notice that your partner has a tendency to *only* do things when they know you're going to be around to see their "sacrifice" or "hard work?". They thrive on recognition. They crave compliments and they won't go out of their way to do anything unless they know someone else is there to witness what they do. If you find that your partner seems to be the type who is constantly fishing for compliments, they are doing it because the narcissist in them is driving those tendencies. Narcissists crave attention. They need it to feed into their egos and belief about their own self-importance. If they can't get it from you through admiration, they will resort to another approach by getting you to feel sorry for them instead. They shift the focus of your attention towards them, their needs, and their so-called "misfortunes". They'll regale you with tales that make you feel sorry for them and feel bad enough for them to shower all your time, and attention is completely devoted to making them "feel better". They will go to any lengths to get the attention they seek, even if they must make up some stories along the way.

- **They Are Obsessed with Power** - They want to be the best of the best. They want to be the smartest person in the room. They want to be the wealthiest person in the room. They want to be the strongest, the bravest, and most popular. They want to be anything that puts them on a pedestal above everyone else. A narcissist *needs* people to look up to them because this is how they develop their self-worth. They want everyone else to feel inferior in their presence, and they want to feel like they are more powerful than you are. They like to surround themselves among people they can feel superior to, like you, for example, if you are a codependent person. They see you as someone they can easily manipulate and control, someone who will give them the attention and validation they seek. If you are dating a narcissist, there is a good chance that your partner thinks they are better than you.

- **They Will Subject You to The Silent Treatment** - Although couples do occasionally use the silent treatment every now and then for as long as anyone can remember, a narcissist will be the one who uses this punishment more than anyone else. Why do they love the silent treatment as a weapon? Because they believe that talking to them is a privilege. They believe they are a gift to everyone around them, and if they withhold their attention or affection, you will be tormented by it. If they feel like punishing you, they will subject you to the silent treatment. Since you are codependent, they know for a fact that this is going to be torture.

- **They Resent Your Success** - A narcissist does not want anyone else to be more successful than they are, and this includes the person they are dating. You know that this is not a healthy relationship that is based on true love when the person who *claims they love you* is the very same person who resents any accomplishment or success you might achieve. In fact, your narcissistic partner might even try to find flaws and faults in your accomplishments and point them out to tear you down and make you feel small. The narcissist takes things a step further by actually shaming and belittling you in public. At any opportunity to lower your self-esteem and make you feel bad, the narcissist will be willing to pounce. The lower your confidence, the more you will learn for validation and approval, and this is exactly what the narcissist wants you to feel. They want you to hang onto every word and continuously come back to them for their approval. Phrases like I was only saying that to help you are commonly uttered by the narcissist, under the guise of doing it for your benefit when really, the only one who is benefitting from this arrangement is them. To make themselves feel better, the narcissist will make everyone else around them feel worse. They'll do everything that they can to make you feel unworthy. This is a dangerous approach when used in a romantic relationship. The narcissist will make their partner believe that they are unworthy of love, and there's no one else out there who will love them the way the narcissists will, just to keep their partner from ever leaving them. They'll destroy their partner's confidence so much that out of fear of being alone or never finding love again, the victim continues to stay in that unhappy and toxic relationship with the narcissist. They will have nothing positive to say about your success or accomplishments because they don't want you to look better than them. They might even treat your success as a direct challenge for them to do better than you and make your success less important. When you are already struggling with codependency, having someone devalue your accomplishments and undermine your success can be a very painful blow to your fragile self-esteem.

- **They Have A Sense of Entitlement** - Does your partner get angry when you say no to them? That is because they feel entitled and they will expect you to give up everything at the drop of a hat if they asked for it. When they know you're codependent, this expectation is magnified, and they will play on your inability to say no by making you feel terrible at the very thought of rejecting their requests. They believe that you are supposed to go out of your way for them since you are in a relationship with them. There is no compromise on their part, all they do is expecting you to be the one who sacrifices everything to make them happy. For example, with a regular couple, your partner might understand if you couldn't bring them lunch they forgot because you were busy at work with your own tasks. A narcissistic partner will get mad at you because they believe their lunch is more important than your job. When there is an obvious pattern of disrespect that is present in your relationship, you know that you are dating a narcissist.

Why Do They Seek to Manipulate You?

Probably the hardest part of being in a relationship with a narcissist is the manipulation that is bound to be part of the relationship. They will use your empathy and love for them against you, one of the most painful forms of betrayal. Why do they seek to manipulate you? *Because they can.* The thing about manipulators is that on some level, they genuinely believe that their way of approaching situations and dealing with people is the right way to go about it. That's often because they are unable to look beyond having their needs met, and that is the only agenda that they care about. They never question themselves because they never see themselves as the problem, to begin with. Manipulators, like the narcissist, will always justify their actions, even when they know they are in the wrong. They will argue their case and make it seem like their negative approach was the only solution to the problem, and therefore they had "no choice" but to do it. They aim to win arguments, rather than come to a mutual consensus, and no matter what you say they will always have a rebuttal against your argument.

Why do they seek to manipulate you when they claim that they "love" you? Because the truth is, the narcissist does not know any other way to operate.

There is a term that is used to describe a tactic that a narcissist would use to manipulate you and make you putty in their hands. That term is called "love bombing". They will shower you with so much love that they literally have you wrapped around their finger. There could be several reasons why they would choose to play mind games on you, and for a narcissist, that reason almost always ends with them getting what they want. If the narcissist knows that asking for something outright is not going to work, then they're going to resort to playing these little games with you because they see it as the only way to achieve their goal. They are very capable of spinning outrageous, pathological lies, smear campaigns, triangulation, and other associated behaviors that defy any reasonable explanation or logic. Manipulative narcissists are often successful in their attempts at deception and control because the tactics that they resort to are ordinary, "normal" and mundane behavioral traits. Easily going unnoticed by anyone who is not active on the lookout for such problematic behavior patterns, and this is precisely what makes them so dangerous. They're in your life, yet you don't realize what's really going on and what they're doing to you.

It can be difficult and very challenging indeed when there is a narcissist in your life. Perhaps the worst part is the way they make you feel insecure about yourself.

Those feelings of insecurity you think you're doing a good job of hiding, hoping that no one notices? The narcissist knows what you're trying to hide. Like many manipulative personality types, they have an uncanny ability to spot those who would make "easy" victims. This, in a way, makes them dangerous predators that have a keen eye for sussing out situations where you may feel uncomfortable or insecure about them. If being criticized in front of others makes you feel insecure, the manipulator is going to take every opportunity they can to belittle you, undermine you, and make fun of you in the presence of others. If making mistakes makes you feel insecure, they will jump at the chance to turn even the simplest mistake and make it seem more disastrous than it really is. When you're already codependent, feeling insecure will make you even more fearful of losing the relationship you have with them because they will reinforce that fear of being alone and losing their affection.

They project such a false sense of self that you would never guess underneath all that bravado, the narcissist can be insecure and full of fear themselves. Oh yes, they are afraid, and their fear is that they will not get their needs met on their own merits. *That* is why they seek to manipulate those around them, especially the ones they perceive to be "weaker" than they are. Like a codependent partner, for example. This is the very basis of narcissism. They have become so separated from the true selves that they subconsciously believe they are "not enough". Instead of dealing with it in a healthy way, they resort to narcissism to make themselves more important. Confront the narcissist about their behavior and you will immediately be met with denial. Yes, even if you were to present them with evidence about their narcissistic tendencies, they'll deny it point-blank and refuse to accept the truth, even if it is literally staring them in the face.

At their deepest core (even though they will never admit it), they do not believe they are enough. Subconsciously, they have created a reality for themselves where they genuinely believe it is them versus the rest of the world. When someone believes they are not worthy of the good stuff, and they are not genuinely connected to who they are, it creates beliefs of lack and scarcity. As a result, they will try to make up for it by convincing themselves they are superior and better than everyone around them. It is a strange coping mechanism that makes no sense to anyone with logic and common sense, but to the narcissist, *this is what makes sense.* Unfortunately, their codependent partner will be on the receiving end of it all.

CHAPTER 5

Codependency And Pathological Loneliness: Why We Stay With Narcissists

The world we live in is a funny thing. We are more connected today than we have ever been in history. The internet has made instantly connecting with family, friends, and loved ones all over the world easy and accessible, something that was not possible several decades ago. Not to mention how nearly everyone these days has at least a smart device of some sort. Some people are fortunate enough to have multiple devices, like mobile phones, tablets, and laptops. When we feel like it, all we need to do is pick up the phone, send a quick text, or make free phone calls over the internet to immediately connect with a loved one. Yet, we are *lonelier* than we have ever been before too. We're so well connected and yet, more people feel alone today than they have ever had before. What is loneliness and why is it so pervasive today?

Understanding Loneliness

Loneliness is subjective. That is because we are all different people who experience emotions in different ways. What one person would describe as loneliness might not be the same as another. For example, you might describe the feeling of loneliness as not having the people you love around you. Someone else might describe loneliness as not feeling connected to the ones they are closest to. The interesting thing is how loneliness is very different from social isolation. A person could have a wide network of people around them and *still* feel lonely and empty. What is even more interesting is how some people who describe themselves as feeling lonely are married to other people. Some people find themselves independent most of the time and prefer to be that way, surrounded only by a few people at any given time. Yet, these people are not lonely.

It is the quality of the relationships that make the biggest difference. This also points out the difference between loneliness and social isolation. The people who prefer to spend most of their time by themselves *choose* social isolation when they feel that they need it. It is a choice because there is some benefit that they receive from it. Introverts, for example, sometimes choose to self-isolate when they feel that they need time alone to recharge and give their energy levels a boost. Introverts are fine being around people, but they may feel drained quickly and don't usually want to be in a social situation for a prolonged period. To recharge their energies, they might need to spend some time alone and once they do get this alone time, they feel refreshed and recharged, able to take on the next social encounter if needed. Introverts are not afraid of interaction if there is an important cause at stake. Introverts are not against social encounters, but they do tend to avoid small talk if the conversation is not going to develop anywhere. That's because they have a limited energy supply to spare and they don't want to drain themselves unnecessarily. For an introvert, being around a lot of people all the time can be overwhelming, and they need this time to themselves to recuperate. Empaths are another example of a group of people who choose to be alone at times. Between juggling their own emotions and the emotions of others, an empath is bound to be emotionally exhausted. Empaths tend to attract people into their lives like magnets because of their gentle and compassionate nature. Being around people is both exhilarating and exhausting for an empath. Alone time becomes a necessity to refuel the emotional gas tank, reset yourself, and gain a sense of balance again. This alone time is necessary to help to prevent burnout. That is social isolation, it is a choice that is made consciously. Loneliness, however, is not by choice.

Why more people experience loneliness today compared to any other period in our history boils down to the internet. With most of our interactions happening online these days, it is easy to feel cut off and disconnected from that human connection. Dating is one example of what would normally be a face-to-face interaction that is happening online a lot more these days through dating apps. Making friends can be done through apps too, the same way dating apps work. Therefore, we are losing a lot of that social connectedness that we used to feel. Sure, it is great that we can do a lot of things these days from the comfort of our own homes, but it can emphasize that feeling of loneliness when you feel too cut off from the rest of the world.

Another reason that creates that sense of loneliness is not being open or vulnerable enough when we are connecting with others. Sometimes, we might not realize that we have our guard up. When there is an invisible wall that is preventing you from being vulnerable, it can make it difficult to feel that connectedness that you yearn for deep inside. Putting on a brave face all the time can be exhausting, both mentally and physically. Somewhere along the way, we somehow developed the belief that showing our vulnerable side is perceived as a sign of weakness. What if we show our vulnerable side, people might take advantage of it? Or worse, we open ourselves up to being hurt. In an attempt to protect our fragile hearts and shield ourselves from hurt, we have become afraid to show any sign of weakness. Sadly, while your intentions may be good, closing yourself off in this way can also prevent you from connecting with people on a deep, meaningful level. You need to show your vulnerable side because as terrifying and scary as it is, you need to know that you can count on some people in your life during the moments when you need it the most. Being in a relationship (any kind of relationship) means pain is sometimes unavoidable, but closing this part of yourself off completely from your partner is not the way to deal with it either. When you can't bring yourself to be open and vulnerable, you are subconsciously holding back part of who you are.

To make matters worse, there are social media channels to contend with. As wonderful as it is, social media is also the source of a lot of unhappiness and relationship problems. Social media is an endless reel of happy, seemingly perfect moments. Everybody wants to show the highlight of their lives and how awesome everything is. Everybody only wants to share their highs, not their lows. Yet, social media has also become a space for cowards and keyboard warriors to criticize, ridicule, and hurt the feelings of other people. It has made us afraid of being open because we don't want to be at the receiving end of criticism and judgment. We are not willing to bare our soul anymore because we're afraid of rejection, thanks to the immense pressure social media has placed upon our subconscious mind to portray perfection.

Loneliness is not a fun feeling. It can rob you of your joy and passion in life. It can cloud your judgment and distract you from your goals. Loneliness is a universal problem, and it is important that we understand the reasons why we feel this way to better understand our codependent tendencies. It can affect you at any age, gender, or status. You can't pretend that it doesn't exist, and there is no magic cure for it either. Not right away, at least. Feeling lonely is something you cannot control, like anxiety and depression. This is a very real and overwhelming problem, and if you don't understand it, it will continue to be a problem that you struggle with every day.

Understanding Why You Feel Alone

We hear the phrase *"you are not alone"* all the time. We might have said it ourselves to try and comfort a friend or a loved one. Yet, does this phrase actually make you feel better? People may tell you that you are not alone, but you still feel alone anyway. What is even more frightening is how loneliness can consume your entire life if you let it. We're all afraid of being lonely, although we may not want to admit it out loud. We don't want other people to know we are afraid of being lonely, and we don't want to admit it to ourselves either. Yet, being codependent is a clear indication that being alone is a terrifying thought. If it wasn't, you wouldn't cling so hard to relationships that might not be the best for you. The fear of being alone is the reason why many find themselves bouncing from one relationship to the next, in hopeful search of happiness.

Here are some reasons why you might experience the loneliness that contributes to your codependent ways:

- **Your Relationships Are Unstable** - This is not specifically romantic relationships alone. It applies to any kind of relationship you have. Friendship, relationships with your family, and even relationships with your colleagues. If the relationships you have in your life are unstable and volatile, it could exacerbate the feeling of loneliness. You become codependent when you finally find someone you can have a genuine connection with. Since the other relationships are unstable, you cling unhealthily to this one special relationship because you're afraid to lose it. Loneliness does not come down to the absence of friends or people in your life. It is a misconception to believe that having friends or people around you means that you will never feel lonely. Loneliness happens when you don't form personal connections that are stable. You only end up feeling unhappy and empty inside because none of your relationships go beyond small talk and meaningless conversation. You hide behind the relationship you depend on because you're afraid that you will never find someone else who understands you this way. Everyone needs stable relationships to feel appreciated, valued, and heard.

- **You Happen to Be An Ambivert** - Loneliness does not always come down to the people in your life. Sometimes, it could be you. The emptiness is a product of who you are. When we think of personality types and how to describe them, we tend to place people into two categories. They are either an extrovert or an introvert. But not everyone can be placed into the introvert or extrovert category. Some people are ambiverts, the ones in between both personality types. When someone feels like they are a mixture of both introversion and extroversion, they are generally known as ambivert. Ambiverts are individuals that favor both elements of introverts and extroverts equally. They like solitude as much as they like socializing. There's no such thing as a pure introvert or a pure extrovert. Even Carl Jung, who was responsible for the theories on introversion and extroversion, believed such a person did not exist. The truth is that introversion and extroversion are a spectrum. For example, if introversion is on the far left of the scale, then extroversion is on the far right. Most people, believe it or not, fall somewhere in the middle. Even the most outgoing social butterflies enjoy time to themselves once in a while. Introverts don't want to be alone all the time either, and they do enjoy the company of the people they love. Since most people are guilty of characterizing themselves incorrectly, they get hung up on the labels. For example, although you prefer to be alone and you think self-isolation is good for you since you believe you are an introvert, being focused on the label leads to neglect. You're neglecting the little extroverted part of yourself that still craves human connection because you've mistakenly believed you're an introvert when you're actually an ambivert. When you only cater to one side of your personality while leaving the other unfulfilled, you're enhancing the loneliness that you feel.

- **You're Striving for Perfectionism -** Some of the loneliest people in the world feel the way that they do because they are striving for a concept that does not exist. They are striving for perfectionism. When you strive for perfectionism, you're afraid of doing anything unless you believe that you can do it flawlessly. This explains why you work extra hard to try and make your codependent relationship work. You're trying to make it perfect, hoping the other person is never going to leave you. You believe that if you never mess up, you're never going to get hurt. Unfortunately, this is rarely ever the case. That feeling of loneliness is never going to go away if you keep chasing a concept that does not exist.

- **Your Expectations Are Too High** - When you're trying to get to know someone new, what are your expectations? Do you expect them to be there for you all the time? Make you laugh? Pick up the phone day or night if you need them? We all harbor secret expectations from the relationships we have in our lives, even if we don't realize it yet. For example, you expect that your best friend is always going to have your back. You expect that your partner is going to love you no matter what. As a codependent, your expectations might be even more unrealistic. When you hold yourself or other people accountable for living up to these unrealistic expectations, it creates deep-seated unhappiness in the relationships. Like perfectionism, no one is going to be able to live up to unrealistic expectations. It is simply not feasible.

Why We Stay With A Narcissist

Codependency is a secondary condition. It is a symptom of a problem that lies much deeper. At the core, those who struggle with codependency often struggle with something else they might not be willing to admit. *They are ashamed.* They suffer from attachment problems too, and this is a byproduct of a trauma that could have occurred in the early stages of their life. If you were growing up around those who were narcissistic and you formed attachments to these individuals, it is very hard to consciously break out of that subconscious cycle unless you know what the problem is. For example, if you were growing up with a parent who was narcissistic, that meant you could not be loved unconditionally. That is because a narcissist is not capable of such love. A child who is exposed to this type of environment will learn to compromise, to be the one who always gives in. They learn to be the "nice" child in hopes that their parents are going to love them a little bit more. They learn to be the people-pleasing child, hoping once again to win the affection of their parents. Little do they realize that their efforts are futile.

When you have been exposed to narcissistic relationships from early on in life, you develop shame and embarrassment. You can't admit to anyone else what is really going on. You can't tell your friends in school that you have a parent who is a narcissist. When you were young, you had no idea what a narcissist is. This kind of relationship is traumatic because it conditions you to believe that the only way to win the love and affections of others is to scan your environment and figure out what you can do to make someone else happy. When you fall short, you feel ashamed, and this feeds into the belief that you are not good enough. It demoralizes you and diminishes your self-confidence. Without realizing it, you have grown to become this person who has become dependent on the approval of others. You have become someone who has developed a fear of being abandoned or alone. No matter how badly you're treated, you would rather keep silent and try to make it better by thinking about what else you can do to please the other person.

You continue to stay with a narcissist because you have lost your sense of self-worth and self-love. Loneliness is a feeling you are all too familiar with. A feeling you have become desperate to avoid. You have developed a perception that you *must* continue sacrificing and always be the one who gives more in the relationship if you want to stop people from leaving you. All those beliefs have manifested into codependency, and at the core of it all, you're doing it to avoid feeling lonely ever again. It is the only way you know how to get rid of this deep, burning pain inside you. Since toxic relationships with narcissists and manipulators are the only types of relationships you know, you continue seeking similar relationships. The problem is, you don't know you're doing this because it is all happening on a subconscious level. In a strange way, you almost feel complete when you're in a relationship with a narcissist.

Being in a relationship with a narcissist is *not your fault.* You have been in this type of relationship for probably years. It takes a lot of strength to walk away from this kind of toxic relationship. The strength that you are working on building for yourself right now. You will eventually be able to leave, but don't blame yourself. You are not weak and you are not worthless, not even a little bit. The fact that you're trying to do something to change shows you're reaching deep inside yourself to find that inner strength already. Some codependents can be very hard on themselves for staying with an abuser and why it took so long before they could walk away. It is not your fault, and these points will illustrate why:

- **They Are Predators** - A narcissist is a manipulator, and like all manipulators, they are predators. They prey on those weaker than them specifically so they can take advantage. They actively seek out those who are weaker for this very reason. They don't love, at least, not in the way that you are hoping for. That is because they are incapable of genuine love when all they think about is themselves.

- **They Fooled You From the Beginning** - A relationship will "love bomb" you from the very start of the relationship. Don't be fooled, though, because they are not doing this out of care for you. This is a strategy. They are purposely giving you the kind of love you probably have never felt before. They love they shower you with could be so intense and one of a kind that your codependent nature did not stand a chance. When you believe that you have found your soulmate, who wouldn't feel ecstatic and in love? The codependent person doesn't know it is a strategy, but the narcissist knows what they are doing every step of the way.

- **They Pull Away on Purpose** - After they have "love bombed" you and made you addicted to those happy feelings of believing that you're in love, they will begin the second phase of their strategy by pulling away. When you feel that loss, you start to crave it. You want it back. You want all those feelings back again because you've become addicted to that kind of love. You want it back so badly you start going out of your way to try and please them, hoping they will turn on the affections again. The narcissist is starving you of the original love on purpose. They know when to come back and give you another hit of love at just the right time. They do this over and over again, shower you with love and then purposely pull away until your withdrawal has become desperation. This is how they keep you hooked on the relationship. Your codependent self will not stand a chance unless you know how to cure yourself of this dependency first.

- **They Contribute to Your Shame** - It's bad enough that you're already feeling low and lacking in self-worth. But does the narcissist care? Of course, they don't. They don't care about anyone but themselves, even if they tell you they love you. Once they realize your codependent nature has made you doubt your abilities and diminished your confidence, they will use that against you. They subtly do things that make you feel even more ashamed of yourself, feeding into your belief that no one can love you unless you're always the one pleasing them. Cruel and hurtful sarcasm is a favorite approach with some narcissists, who enjoy putting their victims down and destroying their self-esteem, all the while disguising their tactics as "a harmless little joke". There's nothing harmless about intentionally making another feel inadequate and bad about themselves. They might even make you feel shame if you were to so much as dare to question their motives. Toxic relationships, like the one you have with a narcissist, will erode your confidence slowly but surely. This is because you are constantly surrounded by people who make you feel like you are never good enough. They make you feel bad about yourself, casting doubt on your abilities, and even make you question whether you are good enough. Being around this all the time will cause wear and tear on your confidence, stripping you of it until eventually, your self-esteem takes a nosedive.

You are the victim in this relationship. The narcissist always knows precisely what they are doing. Everything that they do, they are doing it on purpose. The moves are calculated and everything is geared toward their benefit. Even a non-codependent person could find themselves a victim of the narcissist's whims. A toxic relationship can happen to anyone, even the most intelligent and confident people whom you thought would be too smart to make such poor decisions. There's no telling when and how you might find yourself in a destructive relationship because it often does not start out that way in the beginning. Don't be too hard on yourself, this is not your fault. You were searching for love, like everyone else. This time, the difference is you are going to know how to overcome your codependent tendencies by the time you reach the end of this journey. In some cases, there is hope of fixing the relationship, there comes a point where you need to be willing to walk out the door if nothing changes. That is the only way you will have any power in your hands to do something. You have to be willing to leave your partner if needed.

CHAPTER 6

Identifying Toxic Relationships

Toxic relationships have been mentioned quite a bit. Let's explore the subject in greater detail. Andy Warhol once said: *People should fall in love with their eyes closed.* What did he mean by this? Well, this quote is meant to remind us of the magic that we feel when we start to realize we are falling in love. Falling in love is a wonderful, beautiful, magical experience. That is until the person you end up falling for is not the person you thought they were.

What Is a Toxic Relationship?

It always starts out beautifully. Every relationship is always happy in the beginning, there is no doubt about that. All relationships start out wonderful during the honeymoon phase, and it's no different when a codependent first begin a relationship with a narcissist. However, it won't take long before that quickly fades away into thin air. One of the reasons why this relationship will start off so beautifully is that the codependent will naturally show a lot of love right from the beginning and they shower the narcissist with all the love and energy they have to give. This is what the narcissist wants, and they will keep taking and taking until there is nothing left to give. Sure, the narcissist will put in some effort in the beginning, and once the codependent is convinced they are being loved in return, that is when the tables start to turn. The narcissist will always capitalize on the naivety of the codependent. A toxic relationship is one that can be very damaging because of how it can chip away at your confidence. Being around the constant negativity that toxic people emit will eventually undermine your dignity, affect your self-esteem, and perhaps even warp your personality depending on the relationship's impact.

A Toxic Relationship Could Be With Anyone

It is not just your partner with whom you could form a toxic, codependent relationship. A toxic relationship can exist with *anyone* that you're close to, anyone that takes up space in your life. It could be your spouse, in-laws, sister, brother, uncle, aunt, mother, father, best friend, or even your colleague at work. Everyone has faults, and since nobody is a hundred percent perfect all the time, it becomes a question of identifying when red flags start to show up. Sometimes, people do change. You have probably gone through some major changes in your life that have made you a better person too. Therefore, it is not completely unreasonable to think that a person could change for the better. However, there are also times when you need to stop overlooking the serious issues and see the person for who they are: *A toxic individual.*

There are some parts of a person's personality that they will never be able to change. At least, not without professional help. Unfortunately, these parts are responsible for creating toxicity in the relationship. A healthy relationship is one that epitomizes compassion, freedom, mutual love and respect, listening, security, care, healthy debates instead of arguments, and even healthy disagreements even though both parties may have a difference of opinion. A healthy and happy relationship leaves you feeling energized. You will find none of those in a relationship that is toxic. An unhealthy, toxic, *and codependent* relationship is going to be a zone of negativity, insecurity, power abuse, jealousy, controlling behavior, dishonesty, selfishness, insecurity, low self-esteem, demanding attitudes, criticism, distrust, and the occasional belittling of the person that you are with. A toxic relationship leaves you feeling depleted of energy and in the worst-case scenario, depressed, and perhaps even suffering from anxiety.

The Early Signals

Love can blind us to what is right in front of us. Sometimes, the signs of a toxic relationship were there all along. We simply chose not to see it because we *didn't want* to see it. Relationships can be complicated. When it's good, it can be really great. But when it's bad, it could potentially impact your health physically and emotionally. Nobody wants to find out the heartbreaking truth, that the people whom they have come to love and care so much about are nothing more than toxic for their mental and emotional health. Toxic relationships can quickly bring you down, and if you always let your emotions get in the way of your actions, you could be that toxic relationship.

When you're in love, it is easy to be blind to the fact that your partner is not as emotionally invested in this as you are. Here are some of the early indicators that raise red flag warnings about a toxic relationship, and these are applicable to any kind of relationship you have. These are not exclusive to romantic relationships alone:

- **They Lie More Than They Should** - Is your partner always lying to you and then apologizing for it when you find out? While there is no harm in telling the occasional white lie when it is necessary and if it comes from a place of selflessness. Lying about nearly everything is another matter altogether. It is time to reevaluate how much you can trust your partner if you have caught them in a lie more often than you would like to admit. A healthy relationship needs open communication, honesty, and understanding. If you find that none of these are present in your relationship, then the only conclusion is that you're *not in a healthy relationship* after all.

- **They Are Opinionated** - This is a disguised form of someone who is critical and judgmental. Generally, judgment goes hand in hand with criticism, and if you find this one person in your life is extremely opinionated in a negative way, this could be the red flag you are in the presence of someone who is toxic. Some toxic individuals don't stop at being opinionated either. They become disrespectful too. The disrespectful types are the ones who you need to avoid because they will never be nice to you the way that you deserve. They are often insincere; they bully and they can just be flat out mean and nasty. Disrespectful and opinionated individuals will always be inherently toxic, and this is every reason that you need to stay as far away from them as possible.

- **They Emotionally Manipulate You** - This is a technique they love to fall back on to get what they want from you. When the toxic person in your life is trying to win you over, they have no problems putting you on a pedestal. They will butter you up until they get what they want out of you. The relationship with a toxic personality will never be one that is fair and balanced. It will always be one-sided and in this case, the narcissist is the one who is going to be calling all the shots. By nature, the narcissist wants to have control over everyone in their lives, and the codependent partner is in very real danger of losing themselves in the relationship.

- **They Have A Mindset That Is Punitive** - They gloat when they see misfortune fall upon others. They believe that people deserve the bad things that happen to them. If they have an emotional outburst and lash out at you, and then you come back and tell them they hurt your feelings, they will shrug it off and claim you shouldn't have upset them in the first place. If they treat you badly, they have no problems pointing out that you deserve whatever you get. That you somehow brought the punishment upon yourself. This is an absolutely clear sign that this person in your life is toxic, and you need to rid yourself of them right away. If you subject yourself to this kind of behavior long enough, it is going to destroy your confidence and ability to love yourself until there is nothing left. You will come to believe that every bad thing that happens to you is your fault, and this is not true at all.

- **They Don't Take No For An Answer** - A toxic person always wants things done their way, and this means they will not take "no" for an answer. Tell them no and they will try to get you to change your mind anyway by making the same request repeatedly. They will push your boundaries and sometimes go too far. If a person does not respect your boundaries, they are generally abusive too, because there is nothing stopping them. These toxic individuals make it very difficult to have a normal, healthy, and respectful relationship with anyone in their life because they will literally just push all your boundaries and they do not know when to stop. They will keep pestering you to change your mind and wear you down until you agree to their demands, just to have some peace of mind.

- **They're Always Monitoring You** - Do you find it a struggle to live your life the way you did *before* this person came into it? If that person in your life is bugging you all the time, wanting to know your every move, they are invading your sense of privacy. If you're feeling restricted in the movements and decisions you make, you're in a toxic relationship. A manipulative partner is going to be guilty of this since they always have this need to be in control. They get angry if you try to make decisions without them. They get mad at you if you were to do something without consulting them first. If you ask for their opinion and they give it, but you end up doing your own thing anyway, they get mad at you for that too. If maintaining your individuality feels like a struggle in this relationship, that is how you tell this relationship could potentially be toxic.

- **They Are Entitled, Controlling, and Selfish -** The toxic, selfish person genuinely believes everything is all about them, which is what makes them toxic. They have gone beyond the normal level of selfishness, which all of us have a tendency to do. These toxic individuals feel entitled and superior and believe they deserve the best because they are better than everyone else. They only think about themselves, and sometimes don't even feel bad if they have betrayed you to get what they want. If you find yourself in a relationship with them, they will constantly just take from you without giving anything back in return until it drains you. They are entitled, controlling, and selfish, and if you have a relationship with them, they will expect you to do *everything that they want.* They will never let you have your way, and they never make good partners. Control freaks are toxic people because their actions will cause the relationship to worsen the more you progress. The more you give in to their demands, the more they will demand of you. Control freaks must always be in charge and have full control of the situation, and because oftentimes nothing you do will ever be enough, this can lead to the relationship becoming abusive. For example, if they were to tell you that they don't think you look good in red, but then they see you wearing red anyway, they're going to be mad or upset with you for not listening to them. They could start an argument, and being codependent, you'll immediately try to appease them by apologizing and promising not to make them angry ever again. This is not what a healthy relationship looks like.

- **Frequent Arguments and Conflict** - A loving and people-pleasing soul like the codependent is going to eventually feel tired and fatigued when they keep getting hurt. The narcissist will see the codependent as someone they can walk all over because of how loving and accommodating they can be. You should never be willing to put up with a toxic relationship. It could end up hurting more than just your feelings. Arguments, confrontation, and conflict are all things that drain a person considerably, even if they are not a codependent person, and being trapped in this kind of unhealthy dynamic is going to take its toll on the relationship eventually.

- **They Are Chronically Angry** - Emotional outbursts, moodiness, irritability, these are some of the common symptoms you will find in a person who is chronically angry. An angry person is not an emotionally healthy person, and any relationship they find themselves in is going to be toxic because they are angry people all the time. They could be passive-aggressive when you try to confront them and blame everyone except themselves for the things that go wrong in their life. What is even worse is that they use anger to try and control the people around them, especially once they realize that you are codependent enough to hold onto the relationship. If you're tiptoeing around their anger and controlling what you do because you don't want to make them angry, you're not in a healthy relationship.

- **They Are Chronically Sarcastic** - This is nothing more than a disguised form of anger. Something else that is similar to chronic sarcasm is disparaging humor. The toxic person in your life might use one, both, or alternate between the two, but if they are doing either of these, they are toxic people. When a person is toxic, whether they undermine the ones around them or cause physical or emotional harm, there is usually a reason for it. Sarcasm is wit, but with a lot of bitterness and anger behind it. They will always be putting you down but in a "joking" way. There is nothing funny about belittling the people in your life, and you should never have to put up with anyone who is trying to tear your self-confidence down.

- **They Could Be Paranoid and Insecure** - The codependent one is not the only one suffering from insecurity in the relationship. Underneath all their bravado and big-talk, the toxic person is trying to mask their paranoia and insecurity too. They will be suspicious, and nothing you can do will ever be enough to convince them they have nothing to be worried about. This is why they always need you to agree with them and do what they say. It is their way of trying to reassure themselves that they have control of this relationship. They want to know that they have power over you, and they try to seek the reassurance of this power by trying to control aspects of your life as much as possible. It is exhausting trying to convince a paranoid person, which is why the relationship is often toxic right from the beginning and will only get worse over time. It is best to avoid them completely the minute that you spot them. When you don't do what they say, they don't feel good about themselves, and they will blame you for the way that they feel.

- **They Are Predominantly Self-Centered** - Similar to being selfish, these toxic individuals will always take more than they give. They may give once in a while, but only after they feel satisfied that all *their needs* have been met first. On the rare occasion that they do go out of their way to do something for you, it is never a no-strings-attached favor. They will make a big deal out of it and hold it over your head and perhaps even claim a favor in return later by reminding you how they did this one, little thing for you. They may give, but they will never give *selflessly,* and that is the defining difference that makes them toxic. At the back of your mind, you don't feel good about getting any favors from them because you know there will be a price that you have to pay later on.

- **They Have A Need to Always Be On the Offense** - They believe that people will always try to get back at you or take advantage of you. This kind of mindset leads to them becoming individuals who are always on the offense. They believe that you should strike first before someone else has a chance to strike you. In every interaction or transaction they do, they have this need to always have the upper hand. In their mind, this is how they protect themselves from being taken advantage of. However, this kind of mindset will prevent them from ever having a healthy relationship. As a codependent person, if you grew up around someone with this kind of behavior, you might subconsciously find yourself attracted to similar personality types, even though you don't like their behavior. Why do you continue to seek out this type of behavior when you disagree with it? Because it feels familiar and comfortable.

Can You Rid Yourself of These Toxic Personalities?

Yes, there is a way you can detox yourself from these unhealthy personality types. As a codependent, these steps are going to feel very difficult in the beginning, because the biggest obstacle you are trying to overcome is the inherent need to cling to relationships. Toxic people have a way of getting into your head and messing with your confidence. If you let them, they will hold you back because they prevent you from living your life to the fullest. These steps are doable but don't be too discouraged if you find yourself struggling in the beginning. It's not easy for anyone to separate themselves from the relationships that have been in their life for a long time, especially when it involves family members.

To start inching away from these toxic individuals, this is what you need to do:

- **Take A Break from Them** - You're not a bad person if you feel like you could use a break from the relationship once in a while. Toxic personalities are draining, and if you need to give yourself time to think and reflect about what bothers you in the relationship, take a break from them. When you are reflecting on the relationship, think about why you are fighting this hard to hold on to a relationship you know is unhealthy. Do you miss the person when you are away from them? What do you miss most about them? What you are trying to do is gain some clarity about the negatives and positives in the relationship.

- **Create Emotional Distance From Them** - The key to disentangle yourself from toxic relationships is to create some emotional distance from them. As a codependent, you might struggle with this step quite a bit, but it is a necessary part of the recovery process. During your earlier reflection, you can think about how much distance is necessary if this happens to be someone you can't cut out of your life entirely (spouse or family member). You could seek professional help to improve the relationship if this is someone you can't get rid of entirely, but you still need to pull back. You don't have to be cold towards them, but what you can do instead is to give their opinion less weight. In other words, don't care as much about what they think. Maintain your own thoughts, ideas, and independence by caring a little less about their opinion and create this emotional distance by branching out on your own. Try new things without seeking their opinion first.

- **Learn to Accept What Cannot Be Changed -** Some things can be a hard pill to swallow. Like finding out your parent is a toxic person. Every child wants a close, happy relationship with their parents, but sometimes, that is not always the case. Unfortunately, some people are flawed individuals, and nothing much can be done to change that. Getting upset over the things you cannot change is only going to take its toll on you. Your parents or loved one is not going to be affected by how upset you are over their toxic personality. They will keep doing what they do. If you have toxic parents, you are not to be blamed for it. They may have tried to guilt you, embarrass you, or made you believe that you "deserved" the treatment that you got, but that is not true. If your parents are toxic by nature, there is nothing you can do to change that. As much as you want to have that emotional intimacy with them, if it is not possible, the best thing you can do for yourself and your happiness is to let it go. Once you have reached that acceptance, you can begin to pull back as far as you need until you can be happy being independent and free from their controlling ways. Keep your interactions to a minimum, and don't let their opinions define who you are.

- **Consider Your Contribution** - Is your codependent nature doing anything that contributes to this drama in your relationship? Are you guilty of enabling the toxic people because you have been reluctant to let them go? If the answer is yes, then you know what you need to do next. You need to start getting comfortable with the idea that you have to move away from this person. We usually stay in toxic relationships for a reason, and codependency is one of those reasons. Once you start to recognize how you may be perpetuating the problem, you can begin to do something about it.

Toxic relationships will never benefit you in any way. When one person in the relationship is always trying to control you, it is going to wear you down eventually. Nobody should ever be allowed to make you feel like you are not worthy of getting what you want. You have as much right as anyone to go after your dreams and what makes you happy. Your needs matter as much as anyone else's, and you should never allow yourself to believe you are less important. If you continue to let toxic people have control and influence over your life, you will always believe that you *need them* in your life. Even worse, you believe that you are nothing without them. Curing codependency means cutting out the toxicity that surrounds your life, even if it is painful to do so. Ridding yourself of these toxic personalities is a necessary step to overcome your current, distorted view of relationships. You deserve a loving, healthy, and happy relationship, and it is about time you allowed yourself to believe that.

CHAPTER 7

The True Feelings Of An Empath

Being an empath and being codependent are two different things, but they can be connected in some ways. Understanding the difference is going to help everything make a lot more sense if you're struggling to understand whether you're codependent or just very empathetic to the plight of others.

What It Means to Be An Empath

An empath feels emotions more deeply than other people do. As an empath, you can quite literally feel the emotions of others. When they cry, you cry along with them because you can feel all the pain and sadness that is bringing tears to their eyes. Empaths are very impacted by the feelings of others, and this can be both a blessing and a curse. Empathy can be a blessing because it can bring a real sense of comfort. Often, people who are going through a hard time need you to "be" with them, and this does not always mean help them fix a problem.

There's a sense of comfort that comes from knowing someone completely and wholeheartedly understands what you are going through. When you find yourself in those moments where you don't always know what to say or how to act, pause for a minute. There is no "right way" to approach every emotional situation, and that is the beauty of empathy. It allows you to show your support by being there for them. Empathy allows you to become the refuge that the other person needs.

An empath understands what empathy means. Empathy is not a superpower, it is merely the ability to understand someone else's emotions. An empath knows that empathy is a gift, and they use their gifts wisely in the pursuit of helping others. More importantly, they use their gifts to build relationships. Relationships are what life is all about. We've got a relationship with our families, friends, colleagues, partners, spouses, and various other people we may meet as we journey through life. Some relationships mean everything to us, and obviously, we would want to do everything that we can to keep the relationship healthy. Once a relationship has been damaged, it can often be hard to piece back together, sometimes it can't be fixed at all. This is why empathy matters, because it provides you with the knowledge, tools, and skills that you need to foster and nurture these relationships, to keep them healthy and always thriving. Empathy helps you relate to the people closest to you and the people around you. It helps you to understand how you should react and respond to situations in the best possible manner. At its core, empathy is a complicated human emotion. Not everyone has the ability to genuinely walk a mile in someone else's shoes, and this makes an empath a very special person indeed.

What is interesting about empathy is that most people can actually feel it. Everyone has experienced shades of empathy in some way or another. For example, when you feel bad for the poor mailman who has to walk around on a hot day. You empathize with a mother who is struggling to control her naughty toddler in the grocery store. What differentiates an empath from everyone else is that empaths have more emotional sensitivity and intuitiveness than everyone else. Their intuitive nature gives them the ability to quickly tell what someone is feeling without really thinking about it. An empath is able to instinctively read a person's body language without them having to say a word, and this is something the codependent person cannot do. When an empath actively listens to someone tell their story, they are able to take on their pain, their anger, their happiness, or their excitement. An empath is like an emotional sponge that absorbs the feelings of everyone around them, whether they purposely want to or not. An empath tends to feel emotions more strongly than anyone else and identify closely with the world around them. This changes the way they interact with people and their surroundings.

Sometimes, an empath's gifts help them form strong relationships and new friendships with people. Other times, their abilities could leave them feeling anxious, exhausted, and perhaps reckless. In short, empaths are sensitive individuals, and for some empaths, their emotions can get the best of them. Something that an empath share in common with a codependent person is the desire to help others. An empath instantly jumps at the chance to help someone in distress if it means easing their pain, or when they can clearly see how a person's struggles are impacting them. Empaths relate to what others are going through because it's almost as though they are going through it too. An empath feels a strong desire to help them take away their pain, and they offer to help them in any way that they can.

The Advantages Of Being An Empath

Being an empath is a remarkable gift. For one thing, not everyone is able to tap into this intuitive, sensitive power, it is a power that gives you the ability to form some of the strongest relationships, more so than anyone else. When empathy is combined with social skills, it will help transform the way that you relate to the people around you. For a leader to be able to forge good working relationships with their team members, they need to have good social skills about them. For you to maintain healthy, everyday relationships with the people who matter most in your life, you need empathy and good social skills to work with.

Empaths are special people. Of course, being sensitive to emotions does present its own set of challenges, but being an empath is still a gift. As with any gift, it is not a hundred percent perfect all the time. Some of the advantages of being an empath include the following:

- **Empaths Don't Rush Their Decisions** - A codependent person might rush headfirst into making decisions if they believe it is going to please that special person in their life. An empath does the opposite, preferring to assess the situation and plan their next step. Being a planner can be a good thing since it stops you from rushing to make impulsive decisions. Empaths prefer to choose the best course of action with the least resistance since they don't want to add to their emotional burden if they can avoid it. As an empath, you see deep meaning in certain situations and you're able to assess what the emotional outcomes of each possible situation may be. An empath would spend more time planning their next course of action to avoid rushing into a decision.

- **Empaths Are Connected Deeply to Your Loved Ones** - While your life does not revolve entirely around your loved ones the way a codependent would do it, you are still deeply connected to the ones you love in your life. Sometimes, your connection to them is almost telepathic. You can sense when they are upset even before they have had a chance to say something about it. Your intuition when it comes to your loved ones is strong and you tend to follow that implicitly, and as an empath, you pay attention to your intuition more than other people do. You understand the important people in your life in a way that no one else can. When it comes to your loved ones, your intuition is strong. You follow your intuition implicitly because you trust in your gut instinct.

- **People Tend to Love You Because Of Your Kind Nature** - An empath is a gentle, kind, and caring soul because they feel the emotions of others so deeply. They believe in treating everyone with kindness because of how sensitive they are to emotions. As an empath, you would never intentionally hurt someone because you would feel their pain. An empath can empathize even with difficult people and try to see things from their perspective. An empath would do their best to understand the reason behind someone's behavior.

- **Empaths Are Respectful** - You're also a lot more respectful towards people, and this is one of the many reasons why you are much better at developing close personal relationships. Respect is a vital criterion that is needed to form healthy relationships. People are unique individuals, just like you are, and part of cultivating relationships is accepting others and valuing them for who they are, not who you expect them to be. As an empath, you appreciate the people around you for the unique, individual souls that they are.

- **Empaths Are Easily Overwhelmed At Times -** Other people might not understand why you feel so easily overwhelmed at times. The reason you feel this way is because you're more sensitive than other people, and because of their nature, what is considered normal to others might be overwhelming to them. Extreme sensitivity is not an exaggeration. Imagine an emotion that you're feeling right now, like sadness. Now, imagine feeling the intensity of that sadness by ten times more. When every emotion that you feel is magnified, that intense feeling can cause a great deal of stress for someone who is deeply affected by it. Sometimes, you might find it difficult to control your emotions when you are easily overwhelmed too. You might find that you lose control of your emotions far too often, getting emotionally carried away in situations that have no real cause for it. Difficulty controlling emotions will make it hard for you to manage relationships too.

- **Empaths Can Be Quick At Spotting Liars** - Intuition comes in handy when you need to spot a liar in your midst. This is yet another one of the empath's many hidden talents. If you are an empath, you won't have a hard time spotting a lie, since you can intuitively tell when people are trying to hide something from you. Believe it or not, this is a blessing, since it will stop you from putting your trust in the wrong people. People like the narcissist, for example, who is only looking to take advantage of your kind and forgiving nature. As an empath, protecting yourself from manipulative and toxic personalities is crucial to maintaining balance in your emotions and relationships. There is also a very real danger that empaths might get into relationships with toxic personalities and this can be a real breeding ground for self-destruction. The most dangerous thing about a manipulative individual is how much power they have over your emotions, especially if you're an empath. A toxic person can be so powerful that they can inflict feelings of anger and frustration just by being themselves.

How An Empath Is Different From Being Codependent

One of the key differences that separate being an empath from being codependent is that empaths absorb the emotions of others. They take it all in and become part of the other person's emotions. Codependents, on the other hand, tend to feel *responsible* for the emotions of others. When their partner or someone they love has a problem, they believe it is their responsibility to fix it. Where an empath only feels the emotions of others and goes along with it, a codependent *needs* the other person to feel better in order for *them* to feel better. That is why you'll find a codependent struggling to try and "fix" the situation in the hopes of making things better. They can't feel satisfied until they know you're not upset or emotional anymore. An empath, however, will be by your side while you take your time processing your emotions. An empath is not there to fix anything, but they are there to be your shoulder to cry on if you need it.

Unlike the empath, the codependent does not know what to do with all the emotions you are feeling. They feel them and get upset when you are upset, but they don't know how to process that in a healthy way. They don't know what they should do, and it is not surprising to find a codependent lost and floundering when the person they care about is going through a rough patch. When they can't fix the problem the way they hoped they could, they become upset and frustrated. They become impacted by this, and perhaps even thrown off balance because they don't have the same coping mechanisms as an empath. A clear indication that you're dealing with codependency rather than empathy is when you feel the *need* for that person to be OK in order for you to feel better. Your emotional state depends on how the other person is, and that is when it crosses the line into codependency. This is why you will find that codependents will stop at nothing to make the person they are dependent on feel better. This clearly explains why they go the extra mile, bend over backward, forget themselves, abandon who they are, do things they would ordinarily never want to do, and even neglect their own needs for the sake of making the other person feel better. It is because the codependent *can't* feel better unless the other person does. Other key differences that differentiate empaths from codependents include the following:

- **An Empath Understands** - An empath is able to say to someone that they can understand what they are going through. A codependent, however, would feel stressed that you're upset and would tell the person that they want to help them fix things. Codependents struggle to understand that it is not always about "fixing" the problem. A codependent cannot process the idea that sometimes, a person just needs someone to listen to them without doing anything to try and fix the problem. An empath would encourage you to let it all out to better process your emotions, while a codependent would tiptoe around you because they are afraid of triggering another emotional reaction. This happens when someone doesn't know how to react around you unless you're happy. The codependent gets thrown off when the other person is emotionally thrown off. It is different for an empath since their emotional and mental wellbeing is not tied to the other person. This makes them a better option if you are looking for someone to help you work through your emotions. It is not surprising either to find that a lot of empaths get into jobs that offer guidance and counseling for others because this resonates with their nature. An empath ultimately understands that you cannot fix someone's problems all the time, but a codependent can't grasp this same concept.

- **Empaths Are Great Listeners** - An empath is a great listener because they actively listen to what you have to say. When you speak to an empath about what you're feeling, they are listening with an open mind. They don't approach the conversation with the mindset that they need to solve your problems for you, and therefore, they are not busy trying to formulate solutions in their mind while you are trying to talk to them. A codependent is guilty of this. They mean well, but at the same time, this means that the codependent is not a great listener. When they're not actively listening to you, they're not absorbing the things that you say. They're not processing it in the way that they should. An empath understands that it is important to let people have their say. Allowing the other person to talk freely and work through their own problems allows them to come to a solution on their own. This method works really well, and it makes the other person feel better too. But a codependent will try to interrupt and possibly force solutions that they hope are going to work onto others because they are desperate for the other person to feel better. This doesn't make them a bad person. They mean well, they simply don't understand how to go about it the right way.

- **Empaths Understand That They Can't Save Everyone** - An empath knows that they can only do their best to help in the best way they know-how, but they cannot save everyone. An empath understands that all any of us can do is try our best to help, and that is it. Unlike the codependent, who will be desperate to fix you and get frazzled when things don't work according to plan. A key difference between an empath and a codependent here is that an empath understands that they can only provide someone with the tools to help, but they cannot do the work for you. This is something a codependent would struggle to comprehend. A codependent won't be happy merely offering suggestions or advice, and they will try to do the work for you if you let them. Although it is wonderful that they care this much, this is not a healthy approach to take. By doing this, the codependent is unintentionally stifling the growth of the person they care about. They think they are trying to help, but it is not really helping when you don't let the other person solve their own problems. In fact, the codependent could be making the problem worse. If the codependent is always rushing in trying to save the day, the other person might be in danger of relying on that too much until they forget how to independently solve their own troubles. An empath has more freedom in this case because they are unattached from the outcome. A codependent is not.

- **Empaths Can Be Good Conversationalists** - Empaths can be naturally curious people with a keen interest in the lives of others. Their natural curiosity enables them to be good conversationalists. They are curious about the lives of others without wanting to *become part of their lives,* something that the codependent will try to do once they become attached to them. An empath can pay attention to what is being said, and this allows them to ask all the right questions to keep the conversation going. The codependent will be preoccupied trying to figure out how they can meet your needs or what they can do for you that they won't be paying attention as much as the empath will. To encourage others to open up about their lives, empaths like to focus on open-ended questions and when the other person speaks, the empaths immerse themselves at the moment and listen without interruption. The codependent might be guilty of interrupting when they spot a problem in your story because they will be eager to try and fix it. They make a real effort to be present and minimize distractions that take place during a conversation so they can give the other person their full, undivided attention. Until the codependent learns how to take a step back from their need to fix, they won't be capable of deep, meaningful conversation or attentive listening.

- **Empaths Can Set Boundaries** - An empath is still capable of setting boundaries that protect their emotional and mental wellbeing. It is pretty obvious that a codependent struggles with this concept too. A codependent has a hard time saying no when they know that the person they are emotionally intertwined with needs them. A codependent lives in fear of being rejected if they were to say no, and this makes them incapable of setting healthy boundaries. Boundaries require the ability to say no when you need to, something that a codependent clearly struggles with. An empath knows how to set boundaries to avoid getting hurt because taking on someone else's emotions is not easy. Unless you are an empath yourself, it can be difficult to understand how draining this experience can be. The good thing is, empaths know how to set boundaries for what they are willing to put up with, and they stick to it as best they can. Empaths know how to keep and maintain their distance, and this is one of the best things they could do for themselves when it comes to coping with toxic relationships. The inability to set boundaries is the reason codependents struggle and often feel like they are drowning in a toxic relationship with no way to escape. An empath knows that the more space they put between themselves and others, the better they will feel while still maintaining the capacity to help those who need them.

- **A Codependent Does Not Know How to Differentiate Themselves** - This is something that the codependent needs to work on. They don't know how to differentiate themselves from the person they depend on because they have become fused with that person. Their needs become the codependent's needs, their opinions become the codependent's opinions too. A codependent has become this way because they never had the opportunity to figure out who they are. They have probably spent their lives bouncing from one relationship to the next, driven by that fear of being alone. The codependent has forgotten what is important to them and what they are all about. Their lives have become all about the person they have made their dependent, and this is why it is difficult for the codependent to differentiate themselves. An empath is able to do this since the empath can step back and separate themselves from the problems of others. They will understand and be there for you, absorbing your emotions, but the empath does not *become* part of your world or your problems. An empath knows how to listen to themselves, and they know what makes sense for them. Unlike the codependent, the empath is unlikely to neglect their own needs for the sake of trying to help someone else.

- **An Empath Might Have Mood Swings** - Empaths can swing from one extreme mood to another. Empaths could be happy one moment and then become extremely sad the next. Since an empath feels every emotion ten times more intensely, it is only natural that the way they express these emotions or the mood swings they experience may be heightened as well. An empath who is struggling to get a handle on their emotions might inadvertently lash out at the people who are closest to them. Some people find this extremely difficult to be around since there's no telling when the empath's mood is going to shift or change just like that. The codependent, however, would generally mimic the emotions of the people they depend on. This ties back to the problem of not being able to differentiate themselves once again.

CHAPTER 8

Begin Breaking The Codependency Spell

There is power in being independent. There is even *more power* in walking away from an unhealthy relationship. Breaking free of your codependency spell is, in a way, reclaiming your power. A power that you lost long ago when codependency took over the relationship. When you realize that you are going to be perfectly fine on your own, with or without that one relationship, that is going to shift the dynamic completely. Once this happens, *you* are the one wielding all the power, not the person you have become dependent on.

If you are in a toxic relationship with a narcissist or a manipulator of some sort, the power of walking away is going to give you a strength you never saw coming. Once you walk away and realize that not only did you survive, but you're *happier* because of that decision, it is going to empower you. You're going to get stronger, better, and the next time you have to make such a decision in the future, you're not going to hesitate anymore. Why? Because you have reached a point when you finally realize just how empowering it can be to take back your power. You will not let fear rule your life any longer. If you let your life be run by fear, you're always going to be held back and miss the opportunities that come your way. Even though you may be afraid, you must not let them stop you from living your life. Never be afraid to put yourself out there, because you never know what opportunities or new experiences await you.

Finally Breaking Free

At the end of the day, none of us are perfect. That is, after all, what it means to be human. Still, we can learn a lot from our imperfections if we choose to. The fact that you desire to break free of your codependency already shows that you are taking a major step toward a change for the better. You should be *proud* of yourself because not everyone has this kind of strength or genuine desire to want to change. For someone who has come to rely on the presence of others in their lives, branching out on your own can be a scary thought. Change, any kind of change, is always going to be challenging. It takes great strength and courage to adapt and change to your new surroundings and way of life. Breaking free of codependency is no different.

Before you begin any of the steps below, there is one thing you need to do. *You need to forgive yourself.* If you are still beating yourself up over what happened in the past, it is time to stop. Why are you being so hard on yourself? You know deep down that you don't deserve it. Why do you keep punishing yourself? Everyone makes mistakes, we are only human. That is not a reason to continuously punish yourself. Fill your mind with thoughts that lift you up, not wear you down. The inner monologue can be a very dangerous thing and your own worst enemy, and that enemy has no room in your life if you want to rebuild your self-worth again. The easiest way to overcome this is to think to yourself what advice would I give if my friend or loved one was in this exact situation? If you're going to show them love and compassion and advise them with the best of intentions, then you can do the same for yourself. If you firmly believe that other people deserve compassion, then so do you because you're just as worth it if not more.

The decision to break free of codependency is a decision that will change your life in momentous ways. Now that you know toxic people are such a negative influence in your life, you know that it does not make any sense to keep clinging to such an unhealthy relationship, especially if it is not bringing you any kind of happiness. Now, there is more reason than ever to take action and do what is necessary to reclaim your confidence and self-esteem. Poisonous, unhealthy relationships do not have to control you. To finally break out of the loop once and for all, these are the steps you need to start with:

- **Work On Developing Your Emotional Intelligence** - Emotional intelligence is what separates behaving in a manner that is socially acceptable, and behaving in a way that is completely unreasonable. Human emotions are powerful. They have the ability to completely take over your actions and disrupt your thought process. These emotions can be such a strong and mighty force within us that without the proper techniques to control them, we can easily find ourselves overwhelmed and unable to function effectively. Often, we tend to think of intelligence and emotions as two separate elements. Your codependency is ruled by your emotional fear of being alone or abandoned. Those emotions are strong enough to trigger such a reaction from you, and it has impacted the relationships you have in an unhealthy way up to this point. Your emotions are something that you have to contend with every day, and your ability to successfully handle the emotions and process them enough to a point where you understand what you feel and control it so it does not overwhelm you. Emotionally intelligent people maintain their level of happiness by finding balance in their lives. They never lean towards one extreme or the other. They know, for example, that there must be a balance between having people in your life and being independent. They never try to do too much too soon, instead, they take each moment one step at a time, putting one foot in front of the other, making slow and steady progress. Emotionally intelligent individuals are not just perceptive when it comes to assessing emotions, they are equally as perceptive when it comes to determining their own strengths and weaknesses. This is something you are going to need to help you overcome your struggles with codependency. A lot of people are happy to own up to their strengths but hesitate to accept or acknowledge any kind of weakness. Those with high levels of emotional intelligence are not afraid to own up to their weaknesses, and because they're willing to embrace these weaknesses, they are not held back because of it.

- **Conduct A Self-Assessment** - This is one of the core traits of emotional intelligence. In emotional intelligence, it is *self-awareness.* Conducting a self-assessment on the areas of your life where you believe you have become codependent requires self-awareness to get the job done. It is going to require that you reflect inward, and ask some deep, meaningful questions. A common belief among many expert psychologists is that codependency stems from your childhood, but this is not always the case. You would develop codependency as an adult too, and this is why you need to thoroughly examine the aspects of your life where you believe you can't function without that special person by your side. Why do you feel this way? What is causing your fear? What negative experience have you had in the past that has led you to believe you need to rely heavily on this person for comfort? You could have had a wonderful childhood with parents who gave you everything you could want for and more. Then, you become old enough to encounter relationships outside the family, and one of these relationships could have been the one to trigger all your doubts, worries, fears, and anxieties about being alone. Conduct a self-assessment into where your codependency started, how it came about, what triggered it, and the impact it continues to have in your life.

- **Step Back and Take A Break -** Codependency makes you latch on to something because of that psychological fear of being alone. It makes you latch onto someone else to feel fulfilled. But you *don't need anyone to feel fulfilled* because enjoying your one company once in a while is not a bad thing. As a codependent, you probably can't remember the last time when you stepped out on your own. When was the last time you sat down to enjoy a meal on your own? When was the last time you went out for a movie alone? When was the last time you went for a walk in the park alone to get some fresh air? Or simply spent time at home curled up with a hot cup of coffee and a good book to read? If you're struggling to answer, then you know it has been *far too long*. From this point on, it is important to take a break and spend some quality time *with yourself*. It is even more important to take a break from any relationship that is unhealthy. You cannot discover the new version of yourself if you continue to be weighed down by negative relationships that are holding you back. Anything that is negative has no place in your life, no matter how much you may love and care for the person. The time that you spend alone is the only time you get to properly think about what makes you strong and powerful. This is because when you have this time alone for yourself, you have nothing else to focus on *except yourself*. The other people in your life are not around to distract you and you're not preoccupied with figuring out what you can do for them.

- **Find External Support For When You Need It -** External support could be anything or anyone that brings you comfort. It could be people, books, podcasts, coaches, counselors, YouTube videos, group therapy, anything that you feel is a safe outlet for you to let your emotions out when you need to. You are going to struggle in the early stages, and your emotions are very likely going to overwhelm you. You need to prepare some kind of support system in place for when this happens. Being prepared is the key to making this recovery process a success. Think of this external support as part of the resources and tools you need to help you break out of your codependency spell. This kind of support can provide you with the motivation you need to move forward. Yes, motivation is a *very powerful tool* for any kind of recovery process. Without motivation, it is going to be so easy to give up when the going gets tough. There will be many moments along this journey that are going to push you to your breaking point, and without the motivation to keep you going, you might struggle to make it to the finish line.

- **Practice Mindfulness Of the Mind, Body, and Soul** - Paying attention to your negative thoughts can sound like a scary idea. After all, these are the same thoughts that cause so much fear they make you anxious and codependent in the first place. The last thing you want to do is to be focused on them. Yet, mindfulness is one of the necessary tools for your recovery. How does mindfulness help with your anxious thoughts that continue to keep you trapped in the codependent cycle?? By slowing down your brain long enough for you to calm down. Instead of having your thoughts running a marathon up in your mind, by shifting your focus to what is happening at the moment, your brain is forced to slow down and take in all the current stimuli around it. A slower mind is a less anxious mind. Mindfulness will help you overcome the anxiety brought on by excessive thoughts, and like meditation, it's been around for a while. It is only recently it's becoming more mainstream as more people start to realize its incredible benefits. Ask the happiest people out there what's the secret to their happiness, and they'll probably tell you it's no big secret at all. It's mindfulness. Meditation is one way to ease the worries of your life away, but there are other things you can do to be more mindful every day. For example, you could spend some time in nature. It's sad that we've become so busy chasing careers that we don't spend enough time outdoors anymore. Mother Nature is incredible and wondrous. There's nothing quite like being in her presence. Spend time outdoors, feel the warmth of the sun on your skin, notice how a little gust of wind feels as it caresses your face. Paying attention to the tiny little details around you, like the color of the trees and the details of the flowers, it reminds you how beautiful life is.

You could also try going for a walk in the park. When was the last time you took a long walk to clear your head? You can go for a walk anywhere, whether it's in the city or in nature, and while you're on that walk, tune in to your senses. Be mindful and aware of how each step feels and how incredible it is that you're able to walk. Not everyone is lucky enough to experience that and it is an incredible blessing we often take for granted. Mindfulness can even be practiced while you're eating your meals daily. Put away the screens, turn off the TV and take the time instead to enjoy a delicious, nourishing meal. It's a great exercise in mindfulness. Take the time to appreciate the taste and smell of your food as you chew slowly, bring your awareness to the different flavors and textures. Take your time enjoying your food instead of rushing through it and spend a couple of minutes being grateful as you think about how lucky you are to have food on your plate to fill your belly.

- **Use Music As A Soothing Tool** - You listen to music that you love because it makes you feel good. It can do wonders to calm your troubled soul, and this is also an opportunity to practice mindfulness while you are at it. As you are listening to your music, this time, *really listen* and turn it into a mindful experience. Listen to the lyrics, notice the beats, the melodies, the instruments, the tempo. There is a lot you could be observing and paying attention to once you tune in. How do you respond to that music you're listening to? What's happening in your body? Your mind? Is your body moving to the rhythm? Music has the added benefit of soothing your noisy mind, especially calming instrumental music that is specifically to help you relax. There are a lot of ways you can experience music mindfully and just changing the way we pay attention to the things we normally do anyway can turn it into an entirely new experience altogether. Mindfulness is incredible that way.

- **Date Yourself** - It is another way of spending quality time discovering who you are. Date yourself, treat yourself, challenge yourself. Dating yourself is another way of encouraging you to practice self-care. Invest in self-care, and never neglect taking care of yourself. Unlike what today's world may want you to think, you don't have to be busy all the time. Being busy doesn't necessarily mean you're being productive. Likewise, being productive doesn't mean you need to be busy every minute of the day. Trying to do too much at once is how you overwhelm your mind and trigger intense stressful emotions. When you're burned out and worn out, you get even less done so give yourself permission to unwind and relax. Self-care is as important as getting things done because when your health is compromised, you get nothing done. Invest in activities that help you feel energized and happy. The "me time" and the self-care that you practice during these moments of solitude is when you start to appreciate and value who you are. If you're long overdue for some much-needed self-care, consider spending some quality time alone, read a good book during the weekend with a cup of coffee. This is the time to unwind and relax. Go for a massage whenever you're feeling stressed out. An hour of being pampered while someone else soothes your aching muscles can do you a world of good and leave you feeling refreshed. Exercise, because it keeps you healthy, strong, and fit both physically and mentally and be sure to get enough sleep at night. Watch your favorite TV show or movie that is going to make you laugh. Laughter is the best medicine for just about anything. Meditate and relax. Keep a journal for you to express your emotions whenever you feel the need to. Spend time laughing and catching up with family and friends. In fact, all the previous tips that were discussed in the earlier chapters are a form of self-care in one way or another. There's so much you could do to restore balance in your busy life and fully recharge your depleted batteries.

- **Set Boundaries, Because You Must** - This might not be something that you are comfortable doing, but this is something you *must do* from now on to protect yourself from certain relationships in your life. You must be clear on what you are willing and *not willing* to tolerate. Write down your answers, because these will be the impactful starting points that you are going to use to start setting these boundaries for yourself. Boundaries are the only way to break free of unhealthy relationships that weigh you down. If a person does not respect your boundaries, they are generally abusive too because there is nothing stopping them. These toxic individuals make it very difficult to have a normal, healthy, and respectful relationship with anyone in their life because they will literally just push all your boundaries and they do not know when to stop. Avoid forming relationships with them because it is not worth it in any context. As tough as it is, especially with loved ones and family members, you must start setting up boundaries and be firm about it. Protecting yourself and your own self-worth comes first, and you should never allow yourself to be emotionally bullied by a toxic person, no matter who they are. Do not let someone else make you feel that you are unworthy or inferior, this kind of behavior pattern is dangerous. Setting boundaries helps to protect yourself from them because it helps to limit how much influence they will have over your life. Setting boundaries can be in the form of limiting your time with them or finding a support system to help you manage your emotions after each encounter. It would depend on the situation you may be in. Once you have successfully overcome your struggles with codependency, these boundaries should still be in place. They will tell you when it is time to speak up and when it is time to walk away from a certain relationship in the future.

- **Speak Up** - A lot of times, you might fail to communicate your needs and speak up for yourself if you're codependent. You were afraid of losing this person in the past that you didn't want to do anything that would destroy the relationship, even though part of you knew that you couldn't go on like this forever. At the end of the day, you need to value yourself enough to realize that your need should never be neglected. You need to remind yourself that you will not settle for anything less than you deserve, especially if you are in a relationship with a narcissist. If the relationship has no hope of changing even after you have started speaking up about your needs, then there is only one thing left to do. Plan your exit strategy. Leading up to it, you need to start setting boundaries with that person, be firm and decisive. They may push back and retaliate because toxic people always want to be in control of the situation, but you need to be just as firm and say no. Stand your ground and do not give in to their demands any longer.

Love Yourself Enough To Do What Is Right

You know that a codependent relationship is going nowhere, and it is time that you love yourself enough to do something about it. Perhaps you have tried in the past but didn't get to stick it through all the way to the end. This time, it is going to be different. This time, you are going to *love yourself* and that love is going to be strong enough to make a difference. Learn to love yourself and know your worth, and slowly begin building your confidence from there. You need to love yourself, or rather, learn to love yourself again because you are worth it, and the codependency has made you forget who you are and how much you are worth. Every tool that you are learning in this book will get you to that point of loving yourself. However, you still need to shift your mindset away from believing that you are someone who is not worth loving. None of the tools are going to help if you keep clinging on to that kind of thinking. You've had your fill of negativity in your life with the toxic individuals. It is time to put that behind you. Avoid any kind of negative thoughts completely. If what you've got to say about yourself is even remotely negative, stop at once. Don't do it. Don't say anything at all because it's only going to make you feel even worse about yourself. Whenever you catch yourself doing this, make an active effort to turn that thought around into something positive. It'll be tough to do in the beginning, but it gets easier with practice.

Finally, prepare yourself mentally and emotionally for a lot of hard work down the road. There is no shortcut on the road to recovery. You have to put in the time, effort, and energy into the entire process if you want to make it happen. Positive change for the better can only occur once you let it, and along the way, adjustments may need to be made. Toxic relationships put you to the test and push you beyond your limits, but at the end of the day, once you are out of the relationship, you emerge a much stronger and better person because of it.

CHAPTER 9

Steps To Redraw Boundaries And Rebuild Relationships

Relationships are a difficult territory to navigate. Not only that, they can be complicated too. If you want relationships that are both sustainable and healthy, boundaries are something you must bite the bullet and do. Boundaries are an important part of staying mentally healthy, and we don't realize how badly affected we have become because of codependency until we start enforcing these boundaries. Once we see what a difference having boundaries make in our lives, we start to wonder why we didn't do all of this sooner.

Boundaries are the difference between an average relationship and one that is healthy and fulfilling. Boundaries will point out who are the people you should be investing your time in. This will save you a lot of heartbreak and grief in the future when you spend your time and energy on the wrong type of people.

Reasons Why You *Need* To Enforce Boundaries

Crossing someone's line might not seem like a big deal, but you never know the kind of scar you can leave behind each time you do it. When you cross a boundary, you are crossing a person's emotional and mental limits, and this takes a toll on them. They may tell you everything is fine and it's fine, but the truth is that it's *not fine* at all. You've probably been on the receiving end of this yourself if you are a codependent person. How do you feel when someone crosses your boundary? Sure, you brush it off and tell them not to worry about it, but if you were to admit the truth to yourself, you're *not fine* with it.

When you're in a relationship with a narcissist, they will have no problem violating your boundaries. Not only will they push you to your breaking point, but they will take pleasure in it too. They enjoy pushing others to the limits, and they will go to any lengths to do it, including pushing past your boundaries or violating rules to do so. They may resort to behavior which includes intruding on your personal space, taking or borrowing your things without returning them, taking someone else's work and passing it off as their own, breaking promises, appointments, and even negating on agreements that were made. There is no such thing as respecting boundaries in the eyes of the narcissist, simply because they don't care about anyone else except themselves. In some extreme cases where you might be romantically involved with a narcissist, they could even resort to tactics that include sexual abuse or harassment, domestic violence or abuse, and even verbal and emotional abuse. The worst part of it all is some narcissists even take pride in their behavior under the misguided notion of feeling "powerful" when they see someone else suffer at their hands. Without boundaries, you don't stand a chance against them.

Do you think you don't need boundaries in your life to be happy? *Think again.* Boundaries have become a necessity if you are looking to overcome codependency, and the following reasons will explain why:

- **Boundaries Are Connected To Your Emotional Health** - When you set healthy boundaries, it has a direct influence on the state of your emotional health. As a recovering codependent, you want a sense of control and comfort in your relationships, and boundaries can give you that feeling. When you have firm boundaries in place, you know what you want, and how you want to be treated. You know what you are willing to tolerate and what you won't put up with. When you are clear about these aspects, it protects your emotions. It also helps you maintain control of how you feel, and this will help you avoid feeling overwhelmed when you're in the presence of dominating, toxic, and pushy people. The one thing you can be sure of when it comes to your interaction with others is that people can be unpredictable. Sometimes, even the most well-thought-out interactions will not go according to plan. As much as you want to share your entire life with the people you love, that is not going to be a possibility if they happen to be a manipulator. If you let them, they'll trample all over you and drain you of everything that you have. Without proper boundaries, there's no stopping them from taking advantage of you every step of the way. Boundaries matter not just in your romantic relationships, but in any kind of interpersonal relationship you have to maintain a healthy dynamic between you and the other person while protecting your emotional health too. In the case of the manipulator, as soon as you realize what they're trying to do, you need to immediately enforce your boundaries with them, and let them know what you're not willing to put up with.

- **Boundaries Remind You That You Have A Voice** - When you're codependent, it is easy for your voice to be drowned out in the presence of the people closest to you. You've become so accustomed to putting their needs far above your own that you forget you have a voice of your own too. *You are your own master in this world.* You don't need anyone to complete you and you don't need anyone to make your life feel fulfilled. You are more than capable of achieving all of that on your own. If you are trying to break free of a codependent relationship that is toxic, don't give the manipulator what they want by tolerating their behavior any longer. Don't give them the attention they want, and don't give them the satisfaction of knowing you're deeply affected by what they have done. If they choose to treat you this way, let them know point-blank you're not willing to accept this kind of treatment any longer, explain that when they're ready for a proper conversation, you're ready to talk, and then walk away. Since what the manipulator wants is for you to grovel and beg to inflate their own sense of self-importance, you should do the exact opposite of what they expect and take that power away from them. *You matter. Your feelings and emotions matter. You deserve to be loved and understood too.*

- **Practice Self-Respect** - Self-respect includes setting up boundaries and taking a firm stand in saying that no one is allowed to disrespect you or treat you any less than you deserve. Respect your feelings and your emotions. No one has the right to make you unhappy, and once you make self-respect a habit, you will firmly believe this too. Your feelings and your emotions matter just as much as anyone else. If something doesn't feel quite right, you don't have to go through with it, no matter what the manipulator tries to convince you of. Respect your emotions enough to stand firm on your boundaries and say no with anything you're not happily agreeing with. Make yourself happy first before working on making someone else happy. Manipulators will be waiting to pounce on you the moment they realize their boundaries are not strong enough to hold them back, and they'll keep pushing and testing you until you eventually give in to their demands out of sheer frustration or stress. Respect yourself because you owe it to yourself to take care of your mental and emotional wellbeing, and to protect it from anyone who would try to cause you to harm or destroy your self-worth. You need to be specific and direct about the way you feel. It is up to you to make sure that the people in your life are aware of what is acceptable to you and what is not.

- **It Teaches You How To Say NO** - Since saying no is something a lot of people are uncomfortable with, a good exercise to start familiarizing yourself with the concept would be by setting boundaries. Think of boundaries as a stepping stone towards learning how to say no. You do not feel guilty if you have to say no to someone. If they happen to be a narcissist or manipulator, that is even *more reason* not to feel bad about it. Do you think they would feel bad about inconveniencing you for their own benefit? Of course, they do not. They're trying to take advantage of you, and you are well within your rights to say no to them. They do not have any rights to pressure you into deciding or taking an action you're not comfortable with, and when you firmly say no, remember that you don't owe them an explanation. You can make your own decisions, your own choices, and if you choose to say no, go right ahead. Some manipulators will still attempt to push the boundaries and try to persist despite you telling them no, and you're going to have to be firm and stand your ground. Make it politely, but firmly clear that you're not going to change your mind, and you would appreciate it if they could respect your decision. Say no, thank you, and end the conversation there and then. Sometimes, you need to be assertive if someone you know is being too pushy and not respecting your boundaries. You deserve respect, and this is when assertiveness comes into play. Learn to say no when you want to, and more importantly, when you *need* to. It is going to make a lot of difference in your life.

- **It Makes You More Self-Aware** - Self-awareness is one of the core skills of emotional intelligence, and since emotional intelligence is something you are going to be working on as you overcome your codependent tendencies, self-awareness is going to be one of your core strategies to do it. It's easy to get caught up in the whirlwind of romance during the early stages of the relationship. You want to be with your partner every minute of the day if you could. You want to like what they like, do what they do. Anywhere they go, and everything that they do, you want to be a part of it. But here's where you're in danger of becoming too dependent on them. When your life becomes so intertwined with theirs, you make it much easier for them to assert their dominance over you. It is important that you maintain your independence even when you're in a relationship. That you continue to do the things you did before you met your partner. Keep the same circle of friends, maintain the activities you loved to do prior to the relationship, and above all else, never lose the support network of friends and family you had, no matter how much your partner may try to pry you away from that support system. This sense of independence is going to be what you need to help you get back on your feet again once the relationship with the manipulator has ended. Invest in setting aside time to do some soul-searching. This deep, self-reflection will make you come to the realization that you are responsible for your own happiness. With healthy boundaries, you will come to realize that all you ever needed to feel confident and happy as *yourself.* A romantic partnership is great, but we are also more than capable of surviving without one, and this is a realization you will come to once you start practicing self-awareness.

- **Boundaries Teach You To Be Flexible -** What you will come to realize is that boundaries encourage you to develop a mindset that focuses on being flexible, rather than being perfect. Since you can't control everything all the time, you learn the next best thing is to let go of things that are beyond your control and be flexible. The same way others can't force you to say "no" unless you allow them to, you can't force them to feel a certain way about you. When you no longer try to focus on being "perfect" and having everything done according to your liking, your boundaries will teach you how to stop comparing yourself to others, and this is something you should start working on as you begin the transition into this process of learning how to say "no" more often. The comparison will only serve to leave you dissatisfied and unhappy because no matter what it is never going to be enough. Being controlling will leave you miserable in the long run because you're not trying to understand them. You're trying to control them and this strategy does not work, no matter what you try to convince yourself of. Being controlling is going to drive you and your loved ones crazy.

- **They Serve As A Protective Shield** - Boundaries help to limit your unhappiness, and when you live by guidelines, you learn to appreciate and be grateful for what these boundaries can do for you. It teaches you not to care about what the manipulator thinks of you. Life has enough challenges as it is and we certainly do not need toxic personalities and codependency making things more difficult or complicated than they already are. You definitely do not need to live up or concern yourself with the expectations of the narcissist, if you are in a relationship with them. What you should be focusing on is your own expectations first. If you spend your life always factoring in what people are going to think or say about your decisions, the life you live will never truly be your own.

Toxic people will always try to take advantage of someone who is codependent. Be firm, stand your ground, and don't let them push you around, especially once you realize you're in the midst of a toxic personality. You don't have to be friendly and chatty with them, these people are not your friends. They're constantly on the alert for anything that can be used as a weapon against you, so the more you hold back from them, the harder it's going to be. Set firm boundaries in your dealings with them, and each time they threaten to push against your boundaries, don't be afraid to push them right back out in a firm, yet professional tone. Boundaries help to protect your fragile self-esteem, and this is something you absolutely need as a recovering codependent.

Setting boundaries does not mean you are being unkind. It means you are standing up for yourself and taking control of your emotional and mental wellbeing, and your happiness too. Setting boundaries will pave the way for better, happier, healthier relationships in the future, fostering understanding, and a stronger bond.

How to Set Healthy Boundaries

Setting healthy boundaries that protect your self-worth while preserving the relationship is not as complicated as you might think. Now, setting boundaries might be a completely new experience for you because you've probably never done this before. Not as someone who is trying to recover from codependency, at least. Are you ready to start setting some healthy boundaries and transform your relationships? This is how you do it:

- **Know What You Are Worth** - A lot of the time, we stumble in relationships and end up with the wrong kind of relationships because we don't know what we are worth. You need to know what your true value is *before* you start communicating it to somebody else. Boundaries themselves are based on values. When you set the standards for what you would be willing to accept in your life, they need to be based on values. You might not want to admit it, but there are people in your life who treat you poorly. They could be rude, obnoxious, aggressive, bossy, and even though you might not like to be treated this way, it's still a struggle for you to tell them to stop. The problem is we were not taught how to have healthy boundaries, yet these boundaries are so fundamental in ensuring we achieve success with the relationships we have in our lives. This isn't a subject that we could learn in school, it is something we had to figure out along the way and we're still learning. A boundary that is based on values would be, for example, valuing your time. You value your time and you know it is a precious resource. You like to get things done on time and the boundary that you set is you're not willing to tolerate it when someone is chronically late, even though you have told them that they need to be there on time. If they continue to stroll in late to meetings without a care in the world, that's disrespecting the boundary you set based on something you valued, which was your time.

- **You're Not Seeking Control** - You're not looking for control or power in the relationship. You are simply trying to find a balance between drawing the line without appearing bossy or domineering. Some people believe that they don't want to be viewed as controlling and therefore, they believe they should not have any boundaries at all. However, there are those on the other end of the spectrum, who believe that they need boundaries and therefore, they need to control everything the other person does. They want to make sure the people around them are doing what they want them to do. Both these concepts are at opposite ends of the spectrum and the happy middle is where many people struggle to reach. This happy middle is the ability to set boundaries without being controlling.

- **Explain Rather Than Express** - One way to successfully enforce your boundaries without hurting anyone's feelings is to explain yourself rather than express yourself. When you express yourself, there is a possibility of becoming overly emotional. When emotions get in the way, the conversation can quickly take a turn for the worst when harsh, emotional words are at risk of being exchanged. When you explain *why* you need to enforce these boundaries, you have an opportunity to explain it from an emotionally intelligent point of view. When you express yourself, it comes from a place of logic, and this is much better than having an emotional outburst. When you explain yourself calmly and rationally, you are also giving the other person time to process and work through what you are telling them. Expressing yourself slows down your speech rate, and gives you enough time to think about the responses you want to give. This is going to work much better than blurting out the first few thoughts that spring to mind. Talking about *why* you need to set that boundary and what you hope to accomplish with that boundary is going to give you much better progress in this area.

- **Learn to Trust Your Gut** - Instincts are there for a reason, and they are rarely ever wrong. It is time to start learning how to trust your instinct when it comes to decision-making. When you've made a conscious decision about something, trust that you've made the best decision possible for yourself. Trust that you believe this is the best course of action with the information you have to work with and stand by those opinions. If you don't stand firm and set boundaries, other people are going to come in and push their opinions on you, squashing down your inner truth. If you let them, they'll trample all over you and drain you of everything that you have. Without proper boundaries, there's no stopping them from taking advantage of you every step of the way. Boundaries matter in any kind of interpersonal relationship you have to maintain a healthy dynamic between you and the other person. If you don't want your inner truth to be drowned out, then you need these boundaries in your life.

- **Give Consequences** - When someone does something that is not right and you don't speak up about it, you are enabling their negative behavior. When you don't speak up and tell them about the consequences of their actions, you're indirectly a supporter of their bad behavior. It is like teaching children right from wrong. When a child does something wrong, you tell them the consequences of their actions. You explain why what they did is wrong and what will happen if they do it again next time. Some adults need to be reminded of this too. If you don't speak up, they are only going to keep doing it because they think you don't mind. They don't realize that you might be secretly frustrated or resentful towards them.

Don't Worry About the Guilt, It's Normal

Feeling guilty and backpedaling because you think you might have been too harsh with the boundary-setting, especially with family, is normal. In times like those, just remember that you had to do what was best to protect yourself too, especially if their behavior was getting out of hand and affecting you to the point you felt stressed all the time. resist the urge to apologize for having to say "no." Give yourself some time to adjust to the process. It's going to be hard to not feel guilty straight away. To keep feeling positive, you might need a little extra time to take care of yourself and that's okay. If you need it, go ahead and take it. It's hard to turn off the guilt meter in your brain since our emotions don't work like an on-off switch.

Setting boundaries can be difficult and uncomfortable. If you have never done something like this before, you would probably feel drained and tired by the whole experience. Avoid the need to feel like you have to offer an apology or an alternative solution to make it up to them for having to turn them down. No, you don't need to do this for the toxic relationships that you have because you're still giving them the power over you that they want if you resort to this. You don't need to be sorry about prioritizing your needs before anyone else's. It's okay to feel guilty in the beginning because that is completely normal. This is probably the first time you're having to assert yourself in this way and it is going to feel strange and unnatural at first. Setting boundaries is something that takes a lot of effort and work and to continue sticking to them, so stop and take the time needed to give yourself a little love and self-care.

CHAPTER 10

Being Comfortable In Your Own Skin

Have you ever been told that you couldn't do anything? That if you tried you might fail? It doesn't feel good, does it? To be told that we can't do something is like a blow to our confidence. Each time we are made to feel bad about ourselves, our confidence takes a nosedive. If you have been told this often enough, it could be one overlooked reason that contributed to your codependent tendencies.

Before you can become confident, which is one of the requirements for overcoming codependency, you need to be comfortable in your own skin. This is the segway between self-acceptance and self-love. When you have these foundations firmly built, only then will you be able to quickly gain momentum and build the confidence you need to thrive as a happy, independent individual. Learning to love yourself more and become comfortable in your own skin is going to be a major step in your codependency recovery process.

When you learn to be comfortable in your own skin, it can solve a lot of problems. For example, when you're struggling with a lack of self-esteem, learning to be comfortable in your own skin is the answer. As a codependent person, your need for validation is one of the problems. Being comfortable in your own skin is going to fix that too. You need to love yourself enough to know that you are capable of so much more than you give yourself credit for, and you don't need anyone else's validation to tell you that. Loving yourself is the only way you're ever going to have the courage to be brave enough to stand up for yourself. If you don't love yourself, you're sending a clear message to your manipulative partner that you're easily dominated. That you're a pushover. You need to love yourself first and foremost and use the strength of that love to help you say no when you need to without having to feel guilty about it. A person who loves themselves will never allow themselves to be treated with anything less than respect. This is now the person you need to become once again, depending on how much damage to your self-worth the narcissist might have already inflicted.

You Don't Live To Live Up To Someone Else's Expectations

The only expectations that matter is the one you have for yourself. Nobody's expectations should matter more than that, and you don't have to keep trying to live up to other people's unrealistic ideals. Every time you try to meet someone else's expectations, you're self-sabotaging yourself on the inside. You will continue to feel unfulfilled because you keep doing things to please other people instead of pleasing yourself.

You could do everything perfectly and *still*, there will be someone who has some kind of criticism or comment to make. You will never be able to please anyone, and it is time to pull the plug on this behavior once and for all. When you stop caring about what other people think, that is when you start to free yourself from the chains of unhappiness. Yes, people's expectations are the chains that keep weighing you down. If you think about it, can you honestly say that you are happily trying to meet their expectations? If the answer is no, why do you keep putting yourself through that torment?

Let the new version of yourself care a little less about what other people think. You know who you are, what you're worth, and what you're capable of, and you don't have to please other people at the expense of your own happiness. When you're more concerned with seeking approval from others, you're depriving yourself of the opportunity to develop to your fullest potential. The thing is, not everyone is going to agree with what you do, but if it works for you and you're confident it's the right step to take, then the only approval you need is from yourself. Stop worrying so much about what other people think and instead shift the focus to better yourself for your own benefit. Be flexible and adaptable to the situations and circumstances around you. If things don't go as planned, tell yourself that it is OK and make the adjustments accordingly. It will help to minimize a lot of unnecessary stress and worry if you can learn to adapt quickly to your surroundings.

How to Stop Caring About What Other People Think

When you learn not to care anymore about what other people think, there is going to be immense freedom that comes with it. Feeling easily swayed by what other people say only happens when you're lacking confidence and belief in your own abilities. When you truly love yourself, you see the value you have to offer and you're not going to tolerate any more hatred that comes your way. The only people who are going to matter are the people in your inner circle. Caring about what people think is a natural issue that holds a lot of people back, not just the ones who struggle with codependency. We care about what other people think about us because we are worried about being judged, ridiculed, or criticized. For the codependent, they are worried about what the specific people in their life think because they are worried about losing those relationships.

While it is not wrong to take into consideration how someone else might feel or be impacted by your decision, especially if it is someone you love and care about, it does become a problem when you let this rule your life. We spend too much time worrying about making the wrong impression or what others think about us. Do this long enough and we could eventually find themselves withdrawing from social situations altogether. We have allowed the judgments and opinions of others to become so important to us that we repeatedly neglect our own needs and wants in favor of conforming with the group. It is human nature to care about what people think about you, but when you allow the opinions of others to start affecting the way you act, react, and think, it becomes a problem. It is going to severely hinder your ability to be comfortable in your own skin and love yourself if you keep this up. Changing yourself and your behavior for the sake of constantly accommodating someone else because you're worried about losing them is no way to live.

You need to stop becoming a people pleaser. Some people, like the codependent, can't help but be people pleasers. They can't help themselves, they want so badly for everyone to like them that they are willing to go through great lengths to achieve that. They are willing to do anything to cling onto a relationship, remember? Even if that means putting up with a lot of unhealthy habits and behaviors. That is a problem. The worst part is that sometimes the people whom you allow to influence your decisions are people you don't even like. Now, that is a very real problem. The codependent struggles with this a lot because they don't want to find themselves alone. They don't want to be the odd one out or the one that does not fit in with any type of social group. When you let the opinions of others affect you, it is going to hold you back from being comfortable in your own skin and loving yourself.

Happiness comes from within, not from the opinion of someone else. Happiness is something that cannot be latched onto an external object or person. The time has come to break out of this habit of placing someone else's opinion above your own. To change your perspective, you must be willing to let go of what other people think. You must let go of the need to please others at the expense of your own needs. You must let go of that desperate need for validation and approval from others.

Ditch the Social Media Addiction

There is a ninety percent chance that you have at least one type of social media account. Most people have several social media accounts registered to their name. Facebook, Instagram, YouTube, Snapchat, Twitter, Tiktok, and the list goes on. There is no denying our devices are extremely useful, especially in today's society where we need information fast and on the go. The problem is, our devices are also intentionally designed to be addictive, and the more time we spend on these devices, the more we continue to compare ourselves to the unrealistic expectations we see in the virtual world.

Social media is designed to be addictive, and we can spend hours on one platform alone without realizing it. Apps are designed to keep you coming back for more, but probably the worst part is, it leads you to believe what you see on social media is the truth. All those happy posts of people you know (and the ones you don't know) living their best life is enough to knock your confidence down to the ground. Everything about our digital life is pulling our attention and our focus away from the things that matter. Like interpersonal relationships, for example. The kind you have in real life instead of in the online world. Social media has blurred the lines between reality and fantasy. We see people we know posting happy, exciting moments on their social feeds and we begin comparing our lives to theirs. The grass always seems greener on the other side the more addicted we become until it eventually leads to severe unhappiness. Ditch the addiction to social media as you work on recovering from codependency. It is not going to do you any favors if you keep comparing your life to the unrealistic life you see online.

If you don't want to abandon social media platforms entirely, what you can do is customize your newsfeed. Adjust your settings until all that you see on your newsfeed is content that aligns with your new goals. Uplifting videos, positive quotes, other people who have overcome codependency and shared their tale online.

Fill your newsfeed with inspiration, content that is going to keep you going. There is more than one way to achieve happiness in life, and when you fill your social media newsfeed with the right kind of content, it is going to change your perception and make you realize living up to someone else's expectations is not your sole purpose in life. Social media is a distraction, and your main focus is going to be you. It should be you. Removing distractions from your life will give you the time and the focus that you need to put things into perspective, and assess where your priorities lie. It is important that you spend a few minutes every day just being with yourself. The more distractions you remove, the better.

Start Meditating and Self-Reflecting

One of the secrets to loving yourself more is mediation. If you want anyone to love you the way that you deserve without the codependency aspect of it all, then you must learn to love yourself. One way to ease into the process is to start meditating. Self-reflection and meditation is a process that can be linked together because there are certain aspects of it which intertwine, such as having to spend a few quiet moments alone just to reconnect with yourself. These two processes give us a chance to reflect on your thoughts and what brings meaning to our life, to better understand what we value most. Meditation is a practice that helps you reconnect and focus on the mental side of things, just like self-reflection does. It is an introspective tool, and possibly the only practice out there that can help you tap into the power that lies within your subconscious mind. By making meditation a regular part of your routine, you develop an awareness of yourself and it gives you a greater sense of connection with the world around you. It brings a sense of inner peace and balance, two qualities that can go a long way towards your self-reflective process because of the mental clarity that you gain from meditation which will help you understand what may be holding you down. This is everything you need and more to start overcoming codependency.

Meditation and self-reflection are important tools that you should be taking advantage of because of the life-changing benefits that it can bring. It is not just about improving yourself internally, but the changes that you are going through will soon manifest itself externally too, improving almost all aspects of your life. One example of a benefit that meditation introduces into your life is the way it can improve your relationship with yourself and others around you. We're often surrounded by far too much negativity in our lives, bombarded with images from social media about ideals of perfection that are often unrealistic and only serve to make us question and doubt ourselves. By using guided meditation to reflect on your life, not only will you rebuild that connection with yourself, but the outward relationships that you have will start to improve as you become more mindful about how you treat others.

Codependency has put a lot of strain on your emotional and physical being. At times, you have probably felt blocked, unable to think clearly, and felt lost about what you should do. Meditation will help you clear away the mental blocks that may have been preventing you from getting the most out of your self-reflective process. Meditation is a process that teaches and trains you how to empty your mind and clear your thoughts, which is exactly what you need. It teaches you to live in the present instead of being caught up in all the noise and busyness of your life. Self-reflection cannot happen if we do not live in the present, taking each moment as it comes and appreciating it for what it is. Meditation is the answer to learning how to slow your thoughts and connect with your surroundings, to consistently learn to check in with yourself and how you are doing. As for self-reflection, it makes you more attuned to your emotions, and this can help with your feelings of self-worth and happiness when you are reflecting upon your life. It helps you to view the world with a renewed perspective, concentrating less on the negative aspects.

Yet another hidden benefit of meditation and why it can be such a useful tool in overcoming codependency is the way that it teaches you discipline. The struggle that a lot of people face is not being able to sit quietly enough or long enough to successfully complete a self-reflective process without getting distracted. This is why meditation can help because it is an exercise in discipline. Meditation is something that requires you to sit alone in a quiet space, uninterrupted for an extended period and once you learn how to block out the noise and focus on your thoughts, you find that self-reflection becomes a much easier process.

Meditation also happens to be a tolerance and patience exercise. It is not always easy to sit in the same spot for a prolonged time without, but if you regularly practice meditation, this soon becomes easier and easier each time you do it. When you can learn to patiently sit in one spot and do what you're supposed to be doing, you can learn to be more patient and not be too hard on yourself when you reflect upon your life. Reflecting upon your life can sometimes lead to instances where you can be too harsh on yourself if things are not happening the way you think that it should be, and by learning how to be patient and tolerant through guided meditation, you will learn how to accept and see situations as they are. Living in the moment makes a big difference because it teaches you to let go of the past and not worry too much about the future because that is something you cannot control. Meditation teaches you to be grateful for the present moment that you are living in, appreciating what is happening right now.

Don't Take Things Personally

Once you learn how to not take things personally, you will find that you become immune. Nothing anyone can do or say is going to have power over you any longer.

You won't feel as hurt or stung by the words they say, and you will come to realize that if they don't treat you the way you deserve and they hurt you, then they have no place in your life. Did you know that people are mirrors? Everything that people say or do is really a reflection of themselves, and it has nothing to do with you personally. In a nutshell, you are a canvas for others to project their perspectives and beliefs. Everybody treats each other this way, even you do. We just don't think about it and most people don't even realize it until it is pointed out to them.

Now, this is the most important part. *You have the power to choose whether you want to accept their projections or not.* That's right, you have the power to *reject* their thoughts and opinions if you wanted to. You can choose to say no to them, and you can choose to walk away from the conversation if they are not giving you the respect that you deserve. Everything in your life comes down to how you look at it. You could be someone who sees problems as a problem, or you could be one of the rare few that sees problems as an opportunity. Break out of the box. Shift your perspective, your future self with thank you for it. There is no need to overthink the things that people say to you. Weigh your options and consider the possibilities, but don't overthink it. Getting caught up in obsessing over the worst-case scenario is never productive or necessary. You could spend hours, days, and weeks agonizing over one remark if you spend too much time thinking about every single thing. When you're overthinking, you're not thinking clearly, and that's never the right frame of mind to make any kind of decision. If you find yourself overthinking and can't seem to break out of the cycle, then you need to put your decision on hold. Pause, take a break, and come back to it again when you've done something to break yourself out of that cycle. Never forget that you are in control of your own beliefs, opinions, and perspectives, and there is no reason you should allow someone else to affect you in that way.

When you learn not to take things personally, you develop immunity that is strong enough to make you realize one thing. At the end of the day, it *truly does not matter* what other people say. If it doesn't make you happy, then it is not worth it.

You Don't Need Other People To Tell You What You Are Worth

You are wonderful. You are terrific. You are fantastic. You are amazing and awesome just the way that you are. Let go of the negative thoughts and comments, they have no place in your life any longer as you recover from codependency. When we hold ourselves back from moving forward, it is because of the negative thoughts that are swimming around in our minds. These thoughts that instill a fear of failure. To break out of the box that's keeping you in your mental prison, you need to erase every negative thought that comes into your mind. The minute that you start to change your thoughts, that change in perspective changes your life. Each time you fixate on a negative thought, in embarrassing past experience, obsess about what you can't change, you're leaving the door wide open for worries and anxiety to come waltzing in. Erase the negative comments and opinions from your mind.

One you love yourself enough, nothing anyone can say to you is going to matter. You will no longer see the need to hold onto relationships that make you unhappy either, and this is where you start rebuilding your life once more. The kind of life you deserve, filled with the healthy relationships that you have yearned for all along. Your self-worth should never be tied to how much you can contribute to a relationship, and once you accept this, you are well on your way to becoming a lot more comfortable in your own skin.

Draw a road map of where you want to see your life several years from now. It's not enough to have your goals written down, you need to draw a roadmap of where you want your life to go. We are built to be goal-pursuing machines. For example, if your goal is to be on the right track to overcoming your codependency six months from now, and hopefully overcome it for good a year from now, you need to create a visual road map of that.

Let this visual road map be your guiding light. The map that reminds you that you don't need to tie your self-worth to anyone else. Something you can see in front of you. Make a map of exactly how you plan to get from Point A to Point B. What is the best way to attain everything that you want and what options are you looking at? Don't stress over creating this roadmap, though, because it will shift and change along the way. Sometimes it could take years before you craft out your perfect roadmap. The best approach would be to take it one step at a time. Instead of

focusing on the entire thing all at once, and overwhelming yourself trying to get it right, focus on how you get to your nearest checkpoint and then the next one, and the next one.

Remember, you don't need to waste your time or energy explaining yourself to others. You could explain until you're blue in the face and people will still believe or think what they want to believe. From this point onwards, only your happiness matters in the end. If people don't love and accept you for who you are, then you know those people have no place in your life. The very best thing you can do to be comfortable in your own skin is to surround yourself with the right kind of people in your life.

CHAPTER 11

Things You Can Do To Help Yourself

Being alone and independent sounds great, but it is not always as easy as it sounds. Believe it or not, even introverts sometimes struggle with being alone. While they may enjoy it most of the time, there could be days when they feel weirdly emotional and stressed, wanting to connect to someone familiar. As a codependent, you are bound to experience those same feelings and emotions. There could be moments when you find you are struggling to come up with something to do to keep yourself busy. When you're trying to break free of your codependency, keeping busy is going to be one of the many strategies that will lead to your success. When you're busy and occupied with things to do, you don't have time to think about how much you're missing someone. You don't have time to dwell on the fact that you're operating alone, and this is crucial during the early stages of your recovery.

The early stages are where you are going to struggle the most with learning to be independent. Feeling empty and having a lack of direction are going to be some of the common emotions you experience. Don't worry, this is all part of the process and perfectly normal. Those who are not codependent struggle with the same challenges every now and then.

Being Alone Is Not A Bad Thing

As we get older, we become more independent. We become less dependent on our parents, on other family members, or other adults. Most of us naturally become independent in many different ways, but for some of us, it can be a little hard. Independence, especially as an adult, is extremely important because its benefits far outweigh any disadvantages there could be. There are many reasons and benefits to becoming independent, and these benefits concern both financial and emotional development. Sometimes, we may not know that we are dependent on others, and if you feel you are in a position where this dependency is constraining, then it is worth taking a step back and evaluating how you want to move forward to become more independent.

Instead of thinking about being alone in a negative context, think of this as a time to rediscover yourself. To nourish the passions you forgot about long ago because you were busy trying to please everyone else. Think of this as a time to find joy and gratitude for the little things in life, and to fall in love with yourself once more. Self-love is not to be confused with narcissism.

That's being in love with yourself, that is a different matter altogether. Self-love is a reminder to yourself that you're good enough the way you are, and you deserve to have good things happen to you too. If you have no problem telling people you love how amazing and incredible they are and how deserving they are of love, why not do the same for yourself? For happiness to exist long-term, self-love needs to be present. Time spent alone is an opportunity to cultivate self-love, something that you need to help you overcome your codependent tendencies. When you learn to love yourself, you don't need to rely on someone else to give you the love you seek.

How do you become more independent? Here are five ways to help you break the chains of dependency one at a time:

- **Start A Journey Of Self-Discovery** - Being around people and being dependent on them sometimes blurs the lines and makes it difficult to figure out who you really are. It will be hard to understand yourself as a person and learn about your own strengths and weaknesses. If you are struggling to figure out who you are and what your purpose is, it will be hard to make decisions that are good for your personal growth and development. In fact, it may be hard to even make a decision on your own, and you feel you need to seek the acceptance, validation, and support from the people you are dependent on. To start learning more about yourself, one thing you can do is to start journaling, even if you have no idea what to write. Start with how you feel, what you did yesterday, or at a particular event, what you liked and what you didn't like. Journaling, whether by writing it down or on a private blog, will allow you to observe and reflect on how you feel. It gives you time to think about the behaviors and actions you're doing that are contributing to your codependent tendencies. Discovering your likes, dislikes, strengths, and weaknesses will help you become more independent. It makes you feel a lot more confident as you slowly come to terms with your strengths and begin rebuilding that belief in yourself once more. Journaling can also help you reflect on your own actions and thoughts, enabling you to trust your own instinct. This in turn helps you know what you want out of life and make decisions that benefit your well-being.

- **Build A Happy Morning Routine** - Every day is a brand-new day, a new chance, and a new opportunity to seize the moment and make it the best that you can. Make it a habit each morning to start it right. Starting things off the right way in the morning is a good way to start. Switch up your routine because doing things repetitively can become mundane after a while, no matter how much you love what you're doing. We all need variety in our lives to keep us on our toes and keep things interesting. Break the monotony if it helps you feel good, try something new, experience something you haven't before, and come back refocused and recharged back on track once more.

- **Stop Seeking Validation From Others** - You don't need anyone else to feel complete, and this is something you will finally realize once you complete that self-discovery journey. A huge problem that is contributing to your dependency tendencies is the need to seek validation or acceptance. This could be from your partner, spouse, family, friends, perhaps even your colleagues, depending on the kind of relationship you have with them. Seeking validation and acceptance from others about your life and plans means that you are leading a life based on *their* choices and their aspirations, not your own. This method is hard to do because your brain has been hard-wired to constantly seek validation. You've become so used to this need for approval that you feel lost when you don't have it. This is a necessary step that you need to take, and you are the only one who can do it. It takes strength and courage, as well as practice, to put a stop to this habit. When you finally break free of this cycle, you will find that you can trust your own mind and emotions. You will start to realize that you know what is best for yourself all along. You were simply too afraid to trust in that gut instinct and intuition before. Seeking validation and permission is not entirely wrong, especially when it comes to important, life-changing decisions that might involve other people. But if these validations and permissions are starting to take over your independence, then there must be a line drawn. Make it a daily practice from now on to be more aware of your own feelings, thoughts, and instincts. Other people will never know what is best for you because *they are not living your life.* They are only a part of your life, but they are not walking in your shoes.

- **Learn to Follow Your Joy** - Struggling to come up with things to do? Ask yourself what is one thing you can do right now that you would find fun and enjoyable? Being independent will be a much easier process if you focus on activities that bring you joy. You don't feel time dragging by when you're feeling happy. Indulge in relaxation techniques like listening to soothing music, enjoying a good aromatherapy massage every now and then, anything that works best for you. Some people might even find doing some sort of sporting activity or going for a run relaxing. Whatever it may be if it helps to soothe your frazzled nerves and release the stress from your body, use it to your advantage. Perhaps by learning to follow your joy, you might rediscover an old love.

- **Learn to Become More Assertive** - There's no doubt that dependency strips you off your assertiveness. The need to seek validation and permission is the root cause of this. Becoming more assertive means saying NO, and also putting your own needs above others. This does not mean that you completely neglect the needs of your loved ones. It is perfectly fine to consider their needs, but not at the expense of your happiness. Consider their needs when it is necessary do so, but you should also remember that you need to think about yourself. You need to value yourself too. Sometimes, your habit of immediately saying yes and jumping at the chance to help others makes you forget that you have needs that must be fulfilled too. To cure yourself of codependency, it is important to embrace the ability to be assertive. Be assertive and focus on yourself. Those who care about your wellbeing will understand and encourage this.

- **Learning To Be Selective About Your Social Circle** - You're not anti-social on purpose. Instead, what this step is trying to teach you is to be selective about who you spend time with. In other words, focus on spending time with quality people who uplift you and make you feel better, a particularly important point to remember if you're coming out of a codependent toxic relationship. Be selective over who you spend your time and energy on, and make each relationship you have meaningful and valuable. Fill your life with genuine people, people that you are happy being around.

- **Be Your Own Emotional Support** - We often turn to other people for emotional support, especially when we feel down and stressed. We tend to do this automatically without thinking about it. For the codependent person, turning to others for support has become an addiction. The codependent person has come to rely on this method so much that they have forgotten how to support themselves. There is absolutely nothing wrong with wanting to turn to the people who give you comfort. In fact, it is a great idea to reach out to people you trust for that familiar connection, and to receive the support that you need to get you through the rough patches. That being said, it is equally important to acknowledge your feelings and be your own source of emotional support in case you can't reach the people you rely on. Develop a self-coping mechanism that helps you stay focused and anchor you when you are feeling emotional until you can get in touch with a loved one again. You could develop several coping mechanisms if it helps. The important thing is to learn to rely on yourself, since this will lessen the codependency and the need to reach out to get support. Sometimes, the best kind of support comes from within. When you emotionally support yourself, you can be more in control with your feelings and you don't need to rely on others to feel happy.

- **Spend Quality Time With Yourself** - Another way to practice more independence is by doing things that you'd normally do with other people, on your own. Have you been wanting to try a new restaurant? Go on your own. Want to see a movie but none of your friends are free to go and watch it with you? Go on your own. The idea here is to plan dates with yourself, and it can be anything from something simple as going on a jog or hike alone, or traveling to a country on your own. Doing these things helps to uncover more facets of yourself, understand yourself better, grow your self-value, and self-esteem and it's also a sign of self-love.

How to Be Comfortable Being Alone

You can learn to be comfortable alone, with or without a relationship. One of the best things about being independent is being comfortable with being alone. Being alone and being lonely are two different things. Dr. Eglantine Julle-Daniere describes these two situations beautifully. Being alone, she notes, is "the physical state of not being with another individual, might it be human or animal," while loneliness is a "psychological state characterized by a distressing experience occurring when one's social relationships are (self-)perceived to be less in quantity and quality than desired." We've been told that time alone is negative, and it can be dangerous. This is why we have been conditioned by society to believe that to be happy, one has to be in a relationship or be married. Or when we misbehaved as a kid, we were given a time out or we were grounded, which meant we were isolated from fun and friends.

We all crave social interaction in some form, and this is why social media is so popular. But these social tools have its limitations. When we feel alone, we rush to fill this void with soft addictions like binge watching a TV series, browsing the internet, or spending time on social media platforms. Being independent also means being comfortable with yourself and not trying to fill this void with unnecessary things to drown it out. Instead, you need to build solitude skills to be more comfortable with being alone.

Here are some simple ways to help you get started on building solitude skills:

- **Looking After Your Health** - Our physical health is very much connected to our emotional health. Taking care of what you see on the outside is a quick way to repair how you feel inside. If you work on your physical health, even by doing something as simple as drinking more water, you'll be boosting your overall happiness. Focusing on your physical health is a fast-track to foster a better relationship with yourself and instill self-love. Start with the simple, easy things like exercising regularly, eating a balanced diet and getting enough sleep. All of this is part learning how to enjoy being on your own.

- **Make Plans For Your Future** - This is your life, and it is time to give some serious thought about what you want to do with the rest of it. You can't plan your future around someone else. You need to plan it *for yourself.* Making plans, whether it's a professional or personal goal, helps set a course for your future. It helps guide you in your decision making, giving you something to focus on in the event you feel lost or confused. It also helps to make you feel more optimistic and hopeful for the days ahead, even if you have to face some of it alone.

- **Strengthen Your Coping Skills** - Life is unpredictable and it comes with a variety of stressors. Knowing how to deal with these stressors is called the skill of coping, and that is a skill worth developing. Think about all those battles you faced and what you did to overcome them. Think about what worked and how it worked for you? Think about using that same mindset with the things that are happening to you now, and it's also a good time to give yourself a pat on the back, and give yourself some credit because you earned it. You became more resilient and stronger because of these experiences.

- **Organize Solo Outings** - Not everything you do has to be done with someone. Take out your planner and find interesting things to do and put them on your calendar. It gives you something to look forward to because anticipation is half the fun. Putting things down on a calendar also helps you follow through. Stay in an Airbnb for the weekend, or go for a pottery class, visit a local festival or farmer's market in a nearby town. Find an amazing art exhibition and go for it. Plan things you've been wanting to try and make it happen.

- **Get Creative** - Have you always wanted to try something new? It doesn't matter that you are not good at it. The point is to try something new and different so you can step out of your comfort zone. Learn to play an instrument, write a short story, learn to paint or start a home improvement project. Even if you don't like it, at least you've tried it. Follow your curiosity, because this is the *best time* to learn and explore who you are as a person.

- **Start Learning How to Cook (If You Don't Already Know)** - Sometimes, a really good meal is all it takes to make ourselves feel better. Instead of reheating a microwave meal or pre-packaged food, get cooking. Prepare a fabulous meal just for one, set the table, light a candle, pour yourself a glass of wine, dress up and sit for a good meal. Savor this moment because you're worth it all by yourself.

- **Become A Volunteer** - Volunteer because you want to help out, not because you want to find yourself. In time, helping someone in need will make you fulfilled. Helping others will undoubtedly make you feel better when you know you have made a difference in someone's life, and it also helps you connect to others while also enjoying this quality time alone. There are many ways to volunteer your time and all it takes is a little research within your neighborhood to find out what you can do, and what feels right for you. Make sure the volunteering needs are a good fit for what you are willing and able to do. Performing a random act of kindness also helps so whenever the opportunity is present, do it.

- **Spending Quality Time In Nature** - It sounds like a cliche, but if you haven't tried it, you must. Take a walk, go on a hike, lounge in your backyard or hang out by the beach. Bask in the sunlight, feel the chill on your skin, taste the rain, hear the crunch of leaves-absorb the sights, sounds and smells of nature. Research has proven that at least thirty minutes once a week in nature can improve symptoms of low blood pressure and depression.

- **Disconnect from Social Media** - Incessantly scrolling through your feed can make you feel stressed, especially with all the events going on in the world right now. Taking a break from social media can help reduce the tendency of comparing yourself to others. The picture-perfect newsfeed, the beautiful photos, the perfect bodies, flawless skin, all of these don't tell the whole story. Pictures can lie and you have no idea if these images and videos you see truly portray how a person feels or if they are just giving you the impression that they are as happy as the pictures say they are. But either way, it's no reflection on you. So take time off, take a deep breath, log off social media even for 24 hours.

- **Give Journaling A Try** - Pour your heart and soul out in a safe place that will only be seen by your eyes. Journaling is remarkably therapeutic, and you never know what hidden gems you might discover within yourself once you open the floodgates to your emotions. Journaling is a great way to help keep you on the right track towards being more mindful. Journaling promotes a state of mindfulness because when you're writing down all that you are feeling, you are acknowledging your thoughts and paying attention to them, really seeing them down on paper for the first time in a way you may not otherwise be able to if they are all jumbled up in your mind. Expressing your emotions, especially the things you may not be comfortable revealing to others just yet, has been known to reduce and lower anxiety and stress levels. Even if the only one seeing the journal is you, you just feel better about letting it all out. Instead of letting your mind wander and your thoughts get out of control, writing them down in a journal will force you to bring them into focus, especially when you ask yourself questions in the journal and then attempt to answer them. You might gain insight into why you have been stuck in the codependency cycle for so long, and what the core problem was all this time.

The journey towards independence is not something that can be obtained quickly. It is a process that takes time and effort, as well as the discipline to see yourself through on all the goals and tasks you set for yourself. In time, you can be the independent person you want to be if you set your mind to it, but the important thing to remember is that it is not going to happen overnight. No matter what you take on in life, if you always make it a point to give it your best, you will always get much better results. That's a promise you can hold on to. Giving a hundred percent in all that you do will eventually lead to greater things in life, even if you fail several times along the way. When you fall down, the only way you stay down is if you don't make the effort to stand up again. The ones who go above and beyond are the ones who almost always become successful. Those who work hard, study hard, and train hard will always get more out of their life than those who take it easy, and that's the motivation you need to start making "do your best" a habit you carry with you all day and every day. Be patient and give yourself time to adjust to the process.

Being alone and by yourself is *not a bad thing,* and it is time we all shifted away from this kind of mindset. Life is busy enough as it is, and we should see alone time as a luxury. The ones who learn to be comfortable being independent will go on to become some of the strongest people around. You can become this strong individual too.

CHAPTER 12

Cultivate A Healthy Relationship

Successful relationships have several things in common. For one thing, they are not based on love alone. You love your partner, spouse, or those few significant people in your life, but there is a lot more work that goes into making that relationship a success.

Communication Is the Ultimate One

The number one factor of a healthy relationship is communication. Great relationships simply cannot exist without it. There is no possible way. A lot of problems can happen simply because two people are not communicating well enough. When there is lack of good communication, misunderstandings occur easily. When misunderstandings happen, they are quickly followed by emotions like frustration, anger, annoyance, irritation, and more. You could be annoyed or even angry when you believe that you were misinformed, while the other person could be frustrated and annoyed that you misunderstood what they were saying.

You need to be comfortable telling the people you love how you feel. If you don't, the relationship is always going to be rocky in some way. A deep, meaningful relationship cannot form if you are always holding back some part of yourself.

Practice Forgiveness

When you love someone, that should matter above everything else. Love should matter more than holding on to grudges or anger. Love should be more important than having the last word. When you claim that you love and care about someone, that should take precedence over any petty argument or disagreement. Nothing is worth butting heads with the people you love, and absolutely nothing is worth holding on to anger for. Remember that each time you disagree, one or both people in the relationship are upset. Feelings get hurt, and perhaps words are exchanged that can never be taken back again. Once a word or sentence has been said, it is out there forever. Sometimes, no apology is sufficient to completely erase the memory and pain from the hurt words spoken.

Believe it or not, struggling with forgiveness is not an uncommon thing. Many people struggle with forgiveness, even though they don't realize it until they have given it some serious thought. Gandhi once said that "forgiveness is something that is attributed to the strong." He was absolutely right about that. Forgiveness is one of the most powerful tools you could possess to make letting go of your ego easier. Not only will you eventually gain the ability to forgive others over time when you let go of your ego, but you'll also learn to forgive yourself. You'll learn acceptance, and you'll learn how to be much happier when you let go of all the anger that resides within you.

If you wanted to, you could forgive someone. That is because you always have a choice, it is simply a matter of whether you want to take that choice or not. Most of the time, when we choose not to forgive immediately, it is because we are still harboring anger in our hearts. If there is one emotion you should learn to let go of quickly, it is anger. If there is one emotion that is present and exists in everyone, it is anger. It is considered one of our core emotions, like happiness. It happens even to the best people. While anger is a natural emotion, it becomes a problem when it happens more frequently than it should, especially in romantic relationships. It becomes an even bigger problem when one or both partners refuse to let go of that anger and move on from it. Have you ever had moments where you recalled an argument or a confrontation you had, and the mere thought of it just makes your blood boil all over again? That's what anger can do. It makes you hold onto grudges, makes it hard to forgive, let go and move on.

Prolonged anger in any relationship, not just the romantic ones, can lead to unhappiness, years of not talking to one another and cause relationships to be ruined over matters which are often not worth it at all. The problem with anger in some people is that they find it hard to let go.

As a core emotion, anger on its own is not that much of a problem. It only becomes a problem when it happens too frequently and we find it difficult to let go. Anger becomes a problem when you find it hard to let go of anger, even over the smallest of issues, and you let this anger simmer and boil within you until you explode once again and lash out at your loved ones. Anger becomes a problem when you find it hard to have a happy, meaningful relationship because you constantly find yourself annoyed, frustrated, disgruntled and perhaps even snappy at even the smallest things. You find yourself feeling frustrated and sometimes depressed because of repressed anger issues which you may not even be aware of. You hold onto grudges for a very long time because of that anger and you could end up going for days or weeks without speaking to your partner because of it. You find it hard to express your anger in healthy ways, preferring to let it bottle up inside you instead which leads to other emotional problems. Other people have told you that you have an anger problem, especially your loved ones. You always are pessimistic and negative because of your anger issues.

Creating a quality relationship can happen when both people in the relationship make it a point to practice forgiveness. It is important to realize that all that stuff you get angry about, the things that you're holding a grudge over, it is not worth it. What is worth it however, is your partner. The person you love. The person who is there for you. That is what matters, not your anger. And it certainly isn't worth it to lose someone you love over anger. When you say you do forgive them, say it and mean it. Don't say it for the sake of being able to say that you told them you could forgive them, and yet you still feel angry at them on the inside. When you understand the people you love and practice empathy, forgiveness is going to be a lot easier to come by. Getting angry is easy. But forgiveness? Well, that's a different story. It takes great inner strength to forgive and be the bigger person, and it is going to take a lot of work, but it will well be worth it. It is a choice that you alone must make. It helps to remind yourself that this is someone you love, and that alone should be enough of a reason for forgiveness.

Forgiveness requires a big heart, empathy, and sympathy. It is not always going to be easy to forgive someone when you feel like they have hurt you deeply, but can it be done? Yes, it can.

Understanding The Five Languages of Love

Loving someone cannot be done passively. Gary Chapman is a relationship therapist who pioneered an excellent concept. This concept was called the *Five Love Languages*, and it involved words of affirmation, physical touch, gifts, quality time and acts of service. This is an excellent habit to start working on together with the people you love in your life that you want to develop these healthy relationships with. The Five Love Languages teach you how to give and receive love with awareness, warmth, and love. It reminds us that love is an active thing, and you need to put in the work for it if you want to make it a success. In his book, Chapman highlights that the five languages of love are words of affirmation gifts, acts of service, physical touch, and quality time spent together.

Practicing the language of love requires you to understand yourself and the person that you are with. Some people might respond better to physical touch as their language of love, while others might prefer acts of service or quality time together. You need to figure out what the love language is with the different people you care about. You would also need to think about what their priorities are, and how to respond to them using the five love languages based on those priorities.

Respect Each Other

This goes without saying. If you don't respect someone, you're unlikely to treat them the way that they deserve. This is because you don't care enough about them to make the effort, and that is the truth. All you have to do is look at the relationships you might have had with a narcissist or a manipulator of some sort. Did they treat you with respect? Probably not. Why not? Because they simply did not care enough to do it. In a relationship, no matter who that relationship is with, if you don't that don't respect each other, you will have a much harder time staying together. Respect is a vital habit towards cultivating the happiness in your relationship that you seek. Each time that you show disrespect towards your partner, friend, family member, or loved one, you are indirectly telling them that you don't accept them for the way that they are. Every person is a unique individual, just like you are, and part of being in a relationship is accepting others and valuing them for who they are. It is not who you expect them to be, it is about appreciating them for the person that they are, strength, weaknesses, and all.

It can be hard for your loved ones to respect you in return if you don't demonstrate that same level of respect for them. It is even more important to be respectful in your relationship when you're arguing with each other. A lot of people prefer not to talk about things because they don't want to risk an argument. In the heat of the moment, words get thrown about and often, these may be words that we later come to regret. It's perfectly understandable to feel this way, and what's going to help you during this situation is to remember to always be respectful towards your partner. After all, this is someone that you love, someone you care for deeply and you would never want to hurt them under any circumstances. It cannot be stressed enough how important it is to be respectful throughout a conversation if you want to keep the peace. Respect goes a long way, and when you make your loved ones feel respected, like their opinions and ideas are valued, you will see just how different the interaction is going to become. Rely on empathy and put yourself in their shoes. If they were speaking to you disrespectfully, would you be inclined to just sit there and continue to listen without feeling any kind of negative emotion towards them? Highly unlikely. In fact, that is the quickest way to turn an argument bad, by being disrespectful to your loved one when you're having a conversation with them, because what you're doing is showing them that you don't care about their feelings at all.

Respect your loved ones. Treat them like they are your equals, and not beneath you in any way.

Be Honest, Open, and Sincere

You need to be able to trust the people that you love in your life. If you don't trust them, that relationship is never going to be healthy. The foundation of a happy relationship cannot be built if one, or both people in that relationship do not fully understand just how valuable sincerity is. What it means to be sincere is that you are always making a choice to act with honesty and truthfulness at all times. That's all it takes. Be honest with yourself, being truthful to who you are, what motivates you, what you value and always choosing to be truthful about it with your partner. This is what sincerity in a relationship means. How do you build a relationship that is based on honesty, openness, and sincerity? By thinking about this old saying: Don't make promises that you can't keep. Making promises to your partner or that special someone in your life feels good. It makes you happy to see the smile on their face, but every time you make a promise that you can't keep, the disappointed leaves a little scar within them that chips away at their trust in you. Broken promises hurt, a lot and each promise that gets broken will make it harder for your people to trust you the next time you make another promise, even when you're sincere about it.

Words alone are not enough to convince your loved ones of your sincerity if there's no action to back it up. Another apt saying which sums it all up nicely is actions speak louder than words. If all you're doing is using words to make your partner feel better but nothing ever gets done, it's the same as making empty promises that you can't keep. Honesty, as cheesy as it sounds, is the best policy. When a lack of honesty, openness, and sincerity exists in a relationship, it creates a distance between you and the ones that you love. People can sense when someone isn't being sincere, no matter how well they think they are hiding that fact. It causes communication problems when two people aren't able to freely express how they feel about each other, and try to cover it up instead with lies and untruths. Hiding things from the people that you love will never bring any benefit, even though you may believe it is for their own good. Once trust has been severed between two people, it is very hard to repair the damage and earn their trust back again.

Another aspect of being open, honest, and sincere is to never do something that is not a hundred percent true to who you are. If you're not entirely comfortable doing or saying something, then don't say it. Even if it may be what your partner wants to hear from you. Sincerity doesn't exist if you're pretending for the sake of making someone else happy. They may be happy, but you won't be, not in the long run especially. If you do something for your partner, it should be because you want to, not because you feel like you're being forced into it. If you're not entirely comfortable doing or saying something, then let your partner know right from the very beginning. They'll understand.

Great relationships are here for a lifetime, and if you want your relationships to last, and to be as healthy and happy as they can be, then you need to place honesty as one of your top priorities.

Appreciate the Ones You Love

It is always nice to feel appreciated. You love it when your loved ones show an unexpected gesture that lets you know they appreciate you. They will love it when you do the same for them, especially when they are least expecting it. You know that you feel grateful for your loved ones and appreciate everything that they do. But do you just say how grateful you are for them? Or do you show them how grateful you are through your actions. Don't wait for them to have to ask for something, just do it. Help them out around the house, make a busy day less stressful, buy them flowers for no reason. That way, when you tell them how grateful you are to have them in your life, there is sincerity in it because it was backed up by actions. Show them in little ways that you appreciate them, and more importantly, remind yourself that you are grateful to have your loved ones in your life.

Knowing you are appreciated in a relationship can go a long way toward strengthening the love and care you have for each other. It is easy to take the ones you love for granted. Never wait until it is too late to let someone know that you love them. You don't need to wait for a special or specific occasion to do it either. You could show appreciation for your loved ones every day if you wanted to.

Solve Problems Together

A healthy relationship is fostered when two people think of ways to work together to solve a problem. They accomplish this by thinking about problems as a *"Us versus the problem"* situation. They don't approach problems as a *"Me versus You"* scenario. You are not butting heads with your loved one. You are trying to work out and overcome the problems you have together, and this should be done as a team. This is not a war, and there is no reason to attack each other. Conflicts tend to make some people uncomfortable, and rather than face the problem head on, some people prefer to avoid it. Or they go about resolving the problem in the wrong way, but butting heads with their loved ones instead of trying to work through it by helping each other come up with solutions. Using this approach might not always be a good thing in a romantic relationship. You risk getting your loved one frustrated at your lack of perceived willingness to resolve the situation, and you will get frustrated too because you're actively trying to avoid conflict and dealing with it in the way that you think is best.

Butting heads, pitting yourself against your loved one, attacking each other instead of attacking the problem, *that is the problem* in the first place. A healthy relationship cannot exist in this context. If you change your tune and approach each problem as *"what can WE do to solve this problem together,"* that mindset alone is going to take away half the troubles you encounter in your relationship. Work together as a team and watch your relationship transform.

Laughter Is Ultimately the Best Medicine

If you can make it a habit to make every moment spent with your loved one a happy one that is full of laughter, that relationship is going to thrive so much more because of it. to use humor to help relieve the tension that is sometimes felt from time to time. Being able to laugh is the bridge that brings people closer together, and having a sense of humor has always been recognized as an important quality to have in a long-term relationship. Humor is merely about the funny things that get said, it is also about the things that you do together. It is about having fun in each other's presence, indulging in activities that make you laugh. A sense of humor helps you see the happier, lighter side of life and revel in it.

Laughter has the power to heal and it can touch a deep emotion within us that no other emotion can. In a romantic relationship context, research conducted by the University of North Carolina revealed that couples who shared laughs together had a much happier relationship because of the closeness that they felt and the support they received from their partner. This can work for any type of relationship, from friends, family, colleagues, and more. A lot of the time, the challenges that we go through in life boils down to our capacity to handle it, the way we perceive it and the relationships that we have in our lives that help us get through it. The stronger the bond you share with your loved ones, the better your ability to communicate and work through issues as a team.

Make It a Point to Spend Time Together

Quality time together is just as essential for the relationship's health as any of the other points above. Keeping in touch is easier than ever, thanks to the magic of technology, but it cannot replace the value you get from spending good old fashioned quality time together with the people you love. The relationships you have in your life are a blessing, and they need to be nurtured without the presence of technology. Yes, we all have busy lives that we lead these days, but it is important to find balance between the two. If you neglect your relationships for everything else, your relationships are going to suffer, no matter how much you love and care for those people in your life.

Spending time together in spite of your busy schedules is not as complicated as it seems. An easy way to do this would be to partake in shared common interest activities. Spend some time doing activities together that you and your loved ones enjoy doing. There are bound to be some things that you have in common. It could be a hobby, sport or activity that you like to do together, a shared passion over food perhaps, or even a favorite TV show that both of you love. Make it a habit to do these things together because it can be great for enhancing your communication skills, especially for activities where you need to work together as a team.

When you do spend time together, it is important to set an expectation that you are not going to be distracted by your mobile devices during this time. Understandably, disconnecting for an entire day or maybe two is not entirely possible for many couples. The key is to find a middle ground that works for both of you by setting expectations. Start by committing to setting aside one hour each day to spend time with each other without your phones, tablets or computers present. Both people in the relationship need to come to an agreement to commit to spending this quality time together, and as it becomes a habit, you can slowly move onto increasing the amount of time spent, provided you're both in agreement with it. If you want people to be a part of your life, you have to *make time* for them to be part of it. It is not going to happen magically, it takes hard work and investment.

CONCLUSION

Thank you for making it through to the end of *Cure Codependency*, let's hope it was informative and able to provide you with all of the tools you need to achieve your goals whatever they may be.

Codependency is an addiction, but the good news is, like all addictions, it can be overcome. You now have the strategies you need to help you get the ball rolling. The first and most important step to initiate any kind of positive change in your life is to have the *willingness* and the desire to want to change. The desire to change because you know you want more from this life than what you're currently settled with.

You *don't* need to rely heavily on another person to make you happy. You are more than enough and you are strong enough to carve out your own path to happiness. A happy, healthy relationship should be the cherry on top of your cake, not the foundation that you're trying to build that cake on. You need to carve out a happy and fulfilling life for yourself *first*. It is the only way you're going to rely on yourself for happiness. Once you learn how to do that, you're well on your way to breaking free of your codependency habit. Hopefully, now you have come to realize that codependency is nothing more than a strategy you used because you thought it was the only way to get your needs met in the relationships you have.

Your feelings and needs are not wrong, and they are just as important as anyone else's. You have every right to speak your mind and express your needs, and once you get comfortable doing it, you'll never go back to becoming codependent again. Once you know that you have it within you to say "no" if you don't feel like doing something, and to say it without feeling guilty, you will never find yourself in a situation where you're codependent ever again. Listen to your own needs and feelings, meet those needs, and watch your relationships start to flourish in a healthy way from now on. You are enough and you are worthy. Believe in yourself and love yourself.

Finally, if you found this book useful in any way, a review on Amazon is always appreciated!

www.ingramcontent.com/pod-product-compliance
Lightning Source LLC
Chambersburg PA
CBHW071826080526
44589CB00012B/934